Paraneoplastic and Cancer Treatment-Related Rheumatic Disorders

Guest Editors

KENNETH J. SCALAPINO, MD
CHARLES R. THOMAS Jr, MD

RHEUMATIC DISEASE CLINICS OF NORTH AMERICA

www.rheumatic.theclinics.com

November 2011 • Volume 37 • Number 4

SAUNDERS an imprint of ELSEVIER, Inc.

W.B. SAUNDERS COMPANY

A Division of Elsevier Inc.

1600 John F. Kennedy Blvd., Suite 1800 • Philadelphia, PA 19103-2899

http://www.theclinics.com

RHEUMATIC DISEASE CLINICS OF NORTH AMERICA Volume 37, Number 4

November 2011 ISSN 0889-857X, ISBN 13: 978-1-4557-1189-5

Editor: Rachel Glover
Developmental Editor: Teia Stone

Rheumatic Disease Clinics of North America (ISSN 0889-857X) is published quarterly by Elsevier Inc., 360 Park Avenue South, New York, NY 10010-1710. Months of issue are February, May, August, and November. Business and editorial offices: 1600 John F. Kennedy Boulevard, Suite 1800, Philadelphia, PA 19103-2899. Periodicals postage paid at New York, NY and additional mailing offices. Subscription prices are USD 305.00 per year for US individuals, USD 534.00 per year for US institutions, USD 150.00 per year for US students and residents, USD 360.00 per year for Canadian individuals, USD 659.00 per year for Canadian institutions, USD 427.00 per year for international individuals, USD 659.00 per year for international institutions, and USD 210.00 per year for Canadian and foreign students/residents. To receive student/resident rate, orders must be accompanied by name of affiliated institution, date of term, and the *signature* of program/residency coordinator on institution letterhead. Orders will be billed at individual rate until proof of status received. Foreign air speed delivery is included in all *Clinics* subscription prices. All prices are subject to change without notice. **POSTMASTER:** Send address changes to *Rheumatic Disease Clinics of North America,* Elsevier Health Sciences Division, Subscription Customer Service, 3251 Riverport Lane, Maryland Heights, MO 63043. **Customer Service: 1-800-654-2452 (US and Canada). From outside of the US and Canada: 314-447-8871. Fax: 314-447-8029. For print support, e-mail: JournalsCustomerService-usa@elsevier.com. For online support, e-mail: JournalsOnline Support-usa@elsevier.com.**

Reprints. For copies of 100 or more of articles in this publication, please contact the Commercial Reprints Department, Elsevier Inc., 360 Park Avenue South, New York, New York, 10010-1710; Tel.: (+1) 212-633-3813, Fax: (+1) 212-462-1935, and E-mail: reprints@elsevier.com.

Rheumatic Disease Clinics of North America is covered in *MEDLINE/PubMed (Index Medicus), Current Contents/Clinical Medicine, Science Citation Index, ISI/BIOMED,* and *EMBASE/Excerpta Medica.*

Printed and bound by CPI Group (UK) Ltd, Croydon, CR0 4YY

Transferred to Digital Print 2011

Contributors

GUEST EDITORS

KENNETH J. SCALAPINO, MD
Rheumatology Section, Portland VA Medical Center; Assistant Professor of Medicine, Oregon Health & Science University, Portland, Oregon

CHARLES R. THOMAS Jr, MD
Department of Radiation Medicine, Oregon Health & Science University, Portland, Oregon

AUTHORS

ROHIT AGGARWAL, MD, MS
Assistant Professor of Medicine, Division of Rheumatology and Clinical Immunology, University of Pittsburgh, Pittsburgh, Pennsylvania

JUDITH F. ASHOURI, MD
Division of Rheumatology, Department of Medicine, University of California, San Francisco; Department of Medicine, San Francisco VA Medical Center, San Francisco, California

DAVID I. DAIKH, MD, PhD
Division of Rheumatology, Department of Medicine, University of California, San Francisco; Department of Medicine, San Francisco VA Medical Center, San Francisco, California

R. SAMUEL HOPKINS, MD
Assistant Professor, Department of Dermatology, Oregon Health & Science University, Portland, Oregon

ALEXANDER JACK, MD
Resident, Department of Dermatology, Oregon Health & Science University, Portland, Oregon

SARAH LIPTON, MD
Rheumatology Fellow, Division of Arthritis and Rheumatic Diseases, Oregon Health & Science University, Portland VA Medical Center, Portland, Oregon

HELEN LIU, MD
Resident, Department of Dermatology, Oregon Health & Science University, Portland, Oregon

HUIFANG LU, MD, PhD
Section of Rheumatology, Department of General Internal Medicine, The University of Texas MD Anderson Cancer Center, Houston, Texas

FÉLIX FERNÁNDEZ MADRID, MD, PhD
Professor of Medicine, Division of Rheumatology, Karmanos Cancer Institute, Wayne State University, Detroit, Michigan

MARIA F. MARENGO, MD
Section of Rheumatology, Department of General Internal Medicine, The University of Texas MD Anderson Cancer Center, Houston, Texas

MARIE-CLAIRE MAROUN, MD
Senior Rheumatology Fellow, Division of Rheumatology, Wayne State University, Detroit, Michigan

CHESTER V. ODDIS, MD
Professor of Medicine, Division of Rheumatology and Clinical Immunology, University of Pittsburgh, Pittsburgh, Pennsylvania

HYON JU PARK, MD
Division of Rheumatology, Department of Medicine, Washington University School of Medicine, St Louis, Missouri

PRABHA RANGANATHAN, MD, MS
Division of Rheumatology, Department of Medicine, Washington University School of Medicine, St Louis, Missouri

PASCALE SCHWAB, MD
Assistant Professor, Division of Arthritis and Rheumatic Diseases, Oregon Health & Science University, Portland VA Medical Center, Portland, Oregon

ANJALI SHAH, MD
Resident, Division of Dermatology, Department of Medicine, Loyola University Medical Center, Maywood, Illinois

MARIA E. SUAREZ ALMAZOR, MD, PhD
Section of Rheumatology, Department of General Internal Medicine, The University of Texas MD Anderson Cancer Center, Houston, Texas

CHRISTIAN A. WAIMANN, MD
Section of Rheumatology, Department of General Internal Medicine, The University of Texas MD Anderson Cancer Center, Houston, Texas

Contents

Primary intraocular lymphoma and melanoma in adults as well as leukemia and retinoblastoma in children may present as idiopathic ocular inflammation and require a high index of suspicion. Retroperitoneal fibrosis may mimic lymphoma or a solid malignancy and poses diagnostic challenges. Regional pain syndromes, such as complex regional pain and carpal tunnel syndromes, may be a manifestation of cancer and amyloidosis respectively. Awareness of these rare mimics may serve in guiding diagnostic investigations.

THE CLINICS ARE NOW AVAILABLE ONLINE!

Access your subscription at:
www.theclinics.com

Preface

Paraneoplastic and Cancer Treatment-Related Rheumatic Disorders

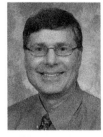
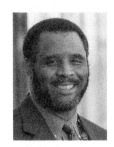

Kenneth J. Scalapino, MD   Charles R. Thomas Jr, MD
Guest Editors

Neoplastic diseases are characterized by a diversity of structural, hematologic, metabolic, immunologic, and biochemical abnormalities producing a wide spectrum of associated symptoms. These features of neoplasm are frequently the target of a growing repertoire of cancer therapies that themselves are capable of producing both local and systemic tissue responses. The diversity of tissues impacted and range of clinical presentations of neoplasm and associated neoplastic therapy are rivaled by few other diseases with the exception of rheumatic disorders and it is therefore common that the differential diagnosis of an occult illness includes diseases from each of these categories. The range of pathophysiologic changes produced by neoplastic disease, neoplastic therapy, and rheumatic disorders is similar in that each can either promote or inhibit cellular proliferation, tissue necrosis and fibrosis, ischemia, or neovascularization and stimulate localized or systemic inflammation. It is therefore not surprising that these processes share not only clinical manifestations, but many laboratory features as well.

Epidemiologic studies of neoplastic and rheumatic disease go further by demonstrating an association between these disorders and support that the shared clinical and laboratory features are more than just chance. Neoplastic tissue can exert a range of influences on the immune system and this immune modulation appears to be just one of several ways in which neoplasm promotes manifestations of rheumatic disease. These findings reinforce the importance of considering neoplasm in patients presenting with the rheumatic symptoms and the value of recognizing the range of autoimmune phenomenon that can develop in the setting of neoplasms and neoplastic therapy.

Rheum Dis Clin N Am 37 (2011) ix–x
doi:10.1016/j.rdc.2011.09.005
0889-857X/11/$ – see front matter **rheumatic.theclinics.com**

This issue of *Rheumatic Disease Clinics of North America* is devoted to exploring the rheumatic manifestations of neoplastic disease and associated therapies. The articles are structured to provide an overview of the association between primary rheumatologic and neoplastic disease followed by an in-depth organ system based discussion of rheumatic manifestations and laboratory features shared by rheumatologic disease, neoplasms, and neoplastic therapy. When possible, these reviews highlight characteristics that help guide the physician in differentiating primary rheumatologic conditions from those secondary to neoplasm and/or neoplastic therapy and in doing so highlight the need for clinical vigilance.

These articles are the work of many talented individuals with expertise across the spectrum of topics including oncology, oncologic-based chemotherapy and radiation therapy, rheumatology, dermatology, and immunology. We would like to thank the contributing authors for their hard work and Elsevier Publishing, Oregon Health & Sciences University, and the Portland VA Medical Center for the continued support.

Kenneth J. Scalapino, MD
Section of Rheumatology
Portland VA Medical Center
3710 SW US Verterans Hospital Road
Portland, OR 97239-2999, USA

Charles R. Thomas Jr, MD
Knight Cancer Institute
Department of Radiation Medicine
Oregon Health & Science University
M/C KPV4, 3181 SW Sam Jackson Park Road
Portland, OR 97239-3098, USA

E-mail addresses:
Kenneth.Scalapino@va.gov (K.J. Scalapino)
thomasch@ohsu.edu (C.R. Thomas)

Rheumatic Manifestations of Cancer

Judith F. Ashouri, MD[a,b], David I. Daikh, MD, PhD[a,b],*

KEYWORDS

- Malignancy • Paraneoplastic manifestation
- Rheumatic disease • Fasciitis • POEMS
- Inflammatory myopathy

Significant overlap in the signs and symptoms of rheumatic disease and occult malignancy requires that cancer be frequently considered in the differential diagnosis of musculoskeletal and rheumatic disease. Musculoskeletal symptoms may be the initial manifestation of malignancy, and their recognition can result in early diagnosis and treatment of a potentially curable malignancy. Patients with both cancer and a rheumatic disorder present an additional challenge in that the development of malignancy may mimic a flare of their rheumatic disease, resulting in delay in the diagnosis and application of an appropriate therapy. In addition, the underlying rheumatic disease, or the immunosuppressive or cytotoxic therapy used to treat that disease, can result in an increased risk of the development of malignancy. Because potent immunosuppressive agents come into more widespread use to treat rheumatic disease, this issue is increasingly important. The neoplastic risks of immunosuppressive agents, which may be the result of diminished tumor surveillance function by the immune system, have been recently reviewed elsewhere and are not considered in detail in this article.[1-3]

Malignancy can result in rheumatic and musculoskeletal disease through several processes. Direct involvement of musculoskeletal structures by primary or metastatic disease leads to local interference with the function of these structures, including connective tissues, muscles, bones, and synovium. Although relatively uncommon in adults, musculoskeletal signs and symptoms predominate in these cases and are directly related to the underlying malignancy. In contrast, a paraneoplastic process refers to the development of organ dysfunction remote from the site of tumor invasion not directly related to the tumor mass itself. Several paraneoplastic syndromes with

^a Division of Rheumatology, Department of Medicine, University of California, San Francisco, 400 Parnassus, San Francisco, CA, USA
^b Department of Medicine, San Francisco VA Medical Center, 4150 Clement Street, San Francisco, CA, USA
* Corresponding author. Division of Rheumatology, Department of Medicine, University of California, San Francisco, 400 Parnassus, San Francisco, CA.
E-mail address: david.daikh@ucsf.edu

Rheum Dis Clin N Am 37 (2011) 489–505
doi:10.1016/j.rdc.2011.09.001
0889-857X/11/$ – see front matter Published by Elsevier Inc.

rheumatic.theclinics.com

rheumatic and/or musculoskeletal manifestations have been described, and most of these result from malignancies that are common in adults. Although cancer can present in a variety of ways, a few specific rheumatic syndromes have been characterized and certainly others that are not reliably categorized as a defined syndrome occur. All these possibilities demand that the clinician be alert to the possibility of an underlying cancer in the patient being evaluated for rheumatic and musculoskeletal disease.

PATHOGENESIS AND TREATMENT OF CANCER-ASSOCIATED RHEUMATIC DISEASE

The development of paraneoplastic disease is thought to be the result of the endocrine effects of the tumor, and a few specific mechanisms of the paraneoplastic disease have been elucidated. For example, most cases of tumor-induced osteomalacia result from increased levels of fibroblast growth factor-23 and/or the *frizzled-4* protein elaborated by the tumor.[4,5] Tumors may also release cytotoxic factors that lead to dysfunction of musculoskeletal or other tissues, resulting in rheumatic symptoms. Tumor antigens can produce hypersensitivity immune responses that lead to secondary tissue damage. Examples of antibody-induced paraneoplastic disease have also been described. For example, patients with teratoma may develop encephalitis as a result of the production of N-methyl-D-aspartate (NMDA) receptor antibodies.[6] In the case of immune-mediated tumor effects, the link between pathogenesis and clinical signs and symptoms of the paraneoplastic disease is similar to that seen in various rheumatic or inflammatory autoimmune diseases that result from inappropriate immune activation. For example, NMDA receptor antibody–induced encephalitis has been recently described in children without teratoma or other malignancy.[7] Further characterization and study of such paraneoplastic processes may lead to improved understanding of the pathogenesis of the underlying malignancy and the rheumatic disease. Pathogenic links between cancer and rheumatic disease that have been identified are noted when relevant. However, this article largely focuses on the clinical manifestations of malignancy-related rheumatic and musculoskeletal disease.

Treatment of paraneoplastic and malignancy-associated rheumatic disease is frequently challenging. In general, these conditions respond poorly to therapies that are typically used to treat rheumatic disease. Their course often parallels the activity of the underlying malignancy. However, many paraneoplastic rheumatic syndromes improve or resolve completely with successful treatment of the underlying malignancy. Conversely, the reappearance of a paraneoplastic rheumatic condition in a patient who has successfully responded to chemotherapy or surgical resection of a malignancy may indicate tumor recurrence. In the absence of a successful cancer therapy, treatment of the associated rheumatic disease is largely symptomatic, although immunosuppressive therapy is commonly attempted and may be helpful for those manifestations that are clearly immune mediated. Corticosteroids in particular may be helpful in cases of inflammatory disease because of their antiinflammatory actions or in cases of hematologic malignancy because they are suppressive and cytotoxic for some hematopoietic cell lines, particularly lymphocytes.[8]

Some paraneoplastic rheumatic conditions manifest with multiple and diverse symptoms that are suggestive of systemic immune-mediated disease. These conditions are discussed as a group. However, many paraneoplastic and malignancy-related conditions become apparent because of the involvement of distinct organ systems. This review of the musculoskeletal and rheumatic manifestations of cancer focus on the disease predominantly involving skin, connective tissues, muscles, joints, and bones.

INVOLVEMENT OF SKIN, CONNECTIVE TISSUE, AND MUSCLE
Fasciitis and Panniculitis

The frequent recognition of skin and subcutaneous tissues as a target of neoplastic disease is likely because, in part, of the visibility of the skin and the dense innervation of these structures, resulting in pain and other sensations when the pathologic condition develops. A large number and variety of individual dermatologic manifestations of cutaneous or internal malignancy are described. Comprehensive descriptions of malignant dermatoses have been published elsewhere.[9,10] However, several paraneoplastic rheumatic syndromes predominantly or prominently involve the skin and subcutaneous tissues and are explained here.

Palmar fasciitis with or without polyarthritis is a rare condition characterized by progressive fibrosis of the hands, resulting in flexion contractures that may suggest the Dupuytren contracture. However, the process is bilateral and usually rapidly progressive. The skin may develop a woody texture suggestive of scleroderma or a more inflammatory appearance that may suggest reflex sympathetic dystrophy.[11–14] Coincident development of carpal tunnel syndrome has been described. Patients with this condition also frequently have polyarticular arthralgias and joint tenderness, which may suggest inflammatory arthritis. The syndrome was first described in association with ovarian cancer, and this tumor association remains the most commonly described.[15–20] However, palmar fasciitis has also been reported in association with several other malignancies, including breast, cervical, bladder, endometrial, gastric, hepatocellular, and lung cancer.[21–27] Although response to steroids has been reported, the condition is usually refractory to therapy; however, successful treatment of the underlying malignancy may improve or halt its progression.

Fasciitis, characterized by inflammation and fibrous thickening of the subcutaneous septa and fascia, occurs in the proximal extremities and occasionally the trunk as a distinct clinical manifestation of autoimmune or infectious disease, which includes eosinophilic fasciitis and the fasciitis-panniculitis syndrome, as well as erythema nodosum.[28] Subcutaneous adipose tissue inflammation, or panniculitis, was first described in association with pancreatic disease by Chiari in 1883.[29] The fasciitis-panniculitis syndrome has been reported occasionally in patients with various forms of malignancy; Hodgkin and non-Hodgkin lymphoma are the most commonly represented, but myeloma and gastric adenocarcinoma have also been reported.[30–32] In this syndrome, subcutaneous inflammation tends to develop in parallel with the progression of the neoplasm. A clinical syndrome of subcutaneous nodules, fat necrosis, and polyarthritis has been well documented in association with acute and chronic pancreatitis and, in particular, with pancreatic cancer.[33–39] When all 3 aspects are present (panniculitis, polyarthritis, and pancreatic disease), it is referred to as PPP.

Pancreatic panniculitis most commonly presents as erythema nodosum, often on the lower extremities but also in the atypical areas involving the trunk and upper extremities. Histopathology of these nodules demonstrates fat necrosis, resulting in the distinct pathologic findings of ghost cells and calcified adipocytes.[40] The arthritis that may develop in these cases seems to most commonly affect the ankles; however, it can lead to long-bone pain as well.[39] The arthropathy seems secondary to periarticular fat necrosis. It is speculated that the panniculitis, as well as the arthropathy, is caused by local autodigestion of subcutaneous or medullary fat from excess systemic levels of digestive pancreatic enzymes such as amylase, lipase, and trypsin.[34,39,41,42] Pancreatic panniculitis may also occur in association with other pancreatic diseases, including pancreas divisum and drug-induced pancreatitis. However, panniculitis may also develop in association with precancerous, intraductal papillary mucinous adenoma, as well as adenocarcinoma of the pancreas.[43] Limited case reports also exist describing erythema nodosum in the setting of parathyroid cancer, lung cancer, and hepatocellular carcinoma without evidence to suggest an underlying connective tissue disease.[44–46] Unlike autoimmune panniculitis, paraneoplastic panniculitis or erythema nodosum characteristically does not respond to nonsteroidal antiinflammatory drugs or glucocorticoid therapy.[47,48] However, similar to other paraneoplastic rheumatologic manifestations of cancer, there may be benefit from treating the underlying cancer. For example, in a patient with hepatocellular carcinoma, who developed erythema nodosum 2 years before the development of tumor, nonsteroidal antiinflammatory drugs and corticosteroids were ineffective in treating the lesions. However, after the tumor was removed, all the skin lesions disappeared without any further treatment.[46] Complete tumor resection is often impossible in pancreatic cancer.

Scleroderma

Sclerodermatous skin changes may also be seen in association with malignancy. However, interpretation of the association between scleroderma and cancer is complicated because some epidemiologic studies have suggested that patients with scleroderma have an increased risk of malignancy[49–53] and because the chemotherapeutic agents used to treat cancer can cause skin changes similar to those seen in patients with scleroderma.[54–56] Nevertheless, a close temporal association between the onset of systemic sclerosis (scleroderma) and cancer has been described in case reports, particularly for breast cancer.[57,58] Other malignancies have also been associated with the onset of scleroderma, including pulmonary, ovarian, and gastrointestinal malignancies.[20,59,60] These cases indicate that at least in some instances, skin fibrosis may be a paraneoplastic process. A group of patients with a close temporal relationship between the onset of scleroderma and the diagnosis of malignancy have been described, who also produce anti-RNA polymerase autoantibodies.[61] RNA polymerase III expression was enhanced in the tumors of these patients, suggesting that RNA polymerase III is a tumor-associated antigen target and, furthermore, that an immune response to this or other autoantigens may be the underlying mechanism of the paraneoplastic development of scleroderma. It remains to be determined whether RNA polymerase antibodies are a predictive biomarker for patients who develop both scleroderma and cancer. This finding has recently been corroborated in a European population.[62]

The Raynaud phenomenon, a common manifestation of scleroderma, can also be an isolated manifestation of occult malignancy and, in some cases, the presenting manifestation.[63–65] The Raynaud phenomenon together with panniculitis has also been described as a cutaneous manifestation of myeloma.[66]

POEMS Syndrome

A group of cutaneous manifestations of plasma cell dyscrasias have been described as part of a distinct paraneoplastic syndrome with rheumatic features called POEMS syndrome, the acronym for polyneuropathy (peripheral neuropathy), organomegaly, endocrinopathy, M-(monoclonal) protein, and skin abnormalities.[67] This syndrome is also called the Crow-Fukase syndrome in recognition of its original descriptors.[68] Multiple myeloma is the most common plasma cell disorder described with this syndrome, but monoclonal gammopathy of undetermined significance, Castleman disease, and plasmacytoma are also seen.[69] Notably, the myelomas described with the POEMS syndrome are usually osteosclerotic, rather than the osteolytic bone lesions typically seen in multiple myeloma. Patients with POEMS syndrome may also develop peripheral edema, anasarca, ascites, or pleural effusion.[70] The most commonly described skin manifestation of POEMS syndrome is hyperpigmentation. However, thickening of the skin, sclerodermatous changes, hypertrichosis, Raynaud phenomenon, whitening of the nails, clubbing, or cutaneous angiomas may present as part of this syndrome.[71] The pathogenesis of POEMS syndrome is unknown. However, the unifying feature of the various manifestations of this rare condition is the presence of a plasma cell dyscrasia, which has led to the hypothesis that cytokines produced by plasma cells are responsible for many of the clinical manifestations of the disease. Tumor necrosis factor α, IL-6, and IL-1β have been implicated, but the most commonly elevated serum cytokine that has been detected in these patients is vascular endothelial growth factor (VEGF). This is also consistent with increased vascularity seen in the involved tissues in POEMS syndrome, which has led some to propose that VEGF has a central role in the disease.[72–74] The anti-VEGF monoclonal antibody bevacizumab has been used to treat patients with POEMS syndrome, with variable success.[75–77]

Inflammatory Myopathies

A well-recognized overlap between rheumatic and paraneoplastic disease occurs in the inflammatory myopathies. Polymyositis and dermatomyositis are characterized by autoimmune inflammatory infiltration of the muscle tissue. This pathologic condition in polymyositis is distinguished by the presence of endomysial inflammation in which multifocal, predominantly CD4$^+$ lymphocytes infiltrate and invade the muscle fibers, whereas the muscle inflammation in dermatomyositis comprises mixed B- and T-cell perivascular, interfascicular, and perifascicular infiltration, resulting in characteristic perifascicular muscle fiber atrophy.[78] In both cases, the muscle inflammation results in myonecrosis and proximal muscle weakness. Dermatomyositis is further distinguished by the presence of 1 or more of a group of characteristic cutaneous manifestations, including Gottron's sign, periorbital heliotrope rash, frequent dilation of periungual capillaries, a thickening and coarsening of the fine dermal structures of the hands (mechanics hands), and erythroderma that may occur on the chest, back and shoulders, face, or generally. Pathologic changes in the skin include dermal perivascular infiltration by CD4$^+$ T cells and capillary dilatation.

An increased incidence of malignancy has been reported with these inflammatory myopathies, but there has been controversy in the literature as to whether the epidemiologic data supporting a cancer association are accurate.[79–81] However, it is now well established that the incidence of malignancy is increased in patients with dermatomyositis, particularly among older patients, in whom the incidence of the associated malignancy may be as high as 25%.[82,83] The pathologic changes seen in cancer-associated dermatomyositis are the same as those observed in the idiopathic autoimmune disease.[84] Most malignancies present within 1 year before or after the diagnosis of inflammatory myopathy.[85] The risk is greatest for middle-aged to elderly patients, aged 45 years or older, although younger patients with the new onset of dermatomyositis also have an increased risk for malignant disease.[83,86] Therefore, older age, as well as poor response to immunosuppressive therapy, should prompt concern for possible malignancy.[82] Age-appropriate cancer screening is indicated for these patients, as well as diagnostic evaluation of any other unexplained signs or symptoms that may signal the presence of occult malignancy, particularly over the first 3 years of the disease.[84] The most commonly described malignancies associated with dermatomyositis are those of the ovaries, gastrointestinal tract, breast, lung, and lymphomas.[78] The evidence of an association of polymyositis and malignancy is less striking than that of dermatomyositis but may also be increased.[80,83,86] In patients with polymyositis, an associated increased incidence of lung and bladder cancers, as well as non-Hodgkin lymphoma, has been reported.[83] The greatest risk of the associated malignancy may be at a younger age in patients with polymyositis.[86]

Much less is known about the association of other types of inflammatory myopathies (ie, inclusion body myositis, dermatomyositis sine myositis, and necrotizing myopathy) with an underlying malignancy. Inclusion body myositis shares some pathologic features with polymyositis and has been reported in association with malignancy, but current evidence does not clearly demonstrate an increased risk of cancer.[87] Dermatomyositis sine myositis, also called amyopathic dermatomyositis, occurs when the skin changes of dermatomyositis are present in the absence of myopathy[88] and, in some cases, may be associated with a paraneoplastic process.[89] However, the number of patients with each type of cancer is too small for a specific association to be made. Nevertheless, the presence of unexplained or atypical myositis should prompt a consideration of coincident malignancy.

Cartilage and Periosteum

Cartilage is infrequently involved in neoplastic processes. The prototypical example is relapsing polychondritis, a condition that involves multiple cartilage sites and results in recurrent inflammation of the nose, ears, trachea, costochondral joints, and other tissues in which type II collagen is present. The inflammatory response is mediated proximally by antibodies to type II collagen.[90,91] Up to one-third of the relapses in patients with polychondritis occur in association with another recognized disease, such as systemic vasculitis; systemic connective tissue diseases, including systemic lupus erythematosus and Sjögren syndrome; or a malignant or premalignant condition.[92–94] An association between relapsing polychondritis and malignancy is well established. Most of the reports of paraneoplastic polychondritis have been in association with myelodysplastic syndrome or hematologic malignancies, but case reports of polychondritis in association with lymphoma, chondrosarcoma, and cancer of lung, bladder, colon, pancreas, and breast have been published.[93,95,96]

Hypertrophic Pulmonary Osteoarthropathy

Hypertrophic pulmonary osteoarthropathy (HPOA) is a well-known example of a cancer-induced paraneoplastic rheumatic disorder. However, it also occurs as a primary condition that usually becomes evident in adolescence and displays autosomal dominant inheritance; sporadic cases of primary disease also occur.[97] HPOA is characterized by proliferative ossifying periostitis of long bones associated with arthritis and clubbing.[98,99] Primary HPOA also frequently includes the presence of thickened skin with prominent skin folds. In contrast to the secondary disease, symptoms are frequently mild with the primary disease. This heritable condition is also referred to as pachydermoperiostosis. Primary HPOA has recently been shown to result from a mutation in the prostaglandin degradation pathway in which a mutation in the HPGD gene results in loss of function of 15-hydroxy-prostaglandin dehydrogenase.[100] Individuals with primary HPOA correspondingly have high urinary levels of prostaglandin E2 (PGE-2).[101] Secondary HPOA occurs in association with a diverse group of inflammatory diseases, most notably intrathoracic infections or inflammatory processes, but also including gastrointestinal or hepatic disease. In addition, HPOA frequently develops in association with malignancy. The most common association is bronchogenic carcinoma but also includes other forms of lung cancer, particularly mesothelioma, and a variety of other malignancies occurring in the thorax or abdomen. HPOA may occur in up to 10% of patients with intrathoracic malignancies. This condition is characterized clinically by a triad of nail clubbing, ossifying periostitis, and periarticular pain, with pain being the cardinal symptom. The periostitis shows a predilection for the ends of long bones. The arthropathy of HPOA generally affects large appendicular joints but also metacarpophalangeal and metatarsophalangeal joints. There may also be surrounding swelling or edema of the soft tissues and occasionally frank synovitis with significant joint tenderness. Arthropathy may also be mild or absent. The predominant symptom is pain in the areas of periostitis, where the skin may be warm, swollen, and tender. Plain radiographs generally reveal the presence of periostitis, frequently with a line of lucency between normal bone and the proliferative periosteum. However, bone pain may occur before the development of significant periostitis. In such cases, a bone scan may be useful in revealing the uptake of radionuclide along the bone margins.[102,103] Given the diversity of conditions in which HPOA occurs, it is particularly challenging to identify the possible pathogenic mechanisms. Because HPOA is frequently associated with intrathoracic processes in which right to left shunting of pulmonary blood flow is present, a leading hypothesis has been that an inactive pulmonary factor is released and activated in the peripheral circulation because of this shunting, leading to the development of HPOA.[104] Another shunt-based hypothesis is that megakaryocytes that normally fragment into platelets in the pulmonary circulation end up in the distal peripheral circulation because of shunting, where they release high levels of platelet-derived growth factor, leading to endothelial activation and perhaps the changes seen in HPOA.[105] However, many of the conditions associated with this syndrome, including most forms of cancer, do not result in right to left shunting, which suggests that other mechanisms must be involved. The major alternative hypothesis is that tumor factors with vascular activity, such as VEGF, are released into the circulation, resulting in the development of at least some of the vascular changes seen in HPOA.[106–108] Another potential clue to the pathogenesis of secondary HPOA has been the dramatic pain reduction observed in a patient with HPOA secondary to lung cancer refractory to narcotic analgesia after treatment with a cyclooxygenase-2 inhibitor, which suggests a role of PGE-2 in the pathogenesis of HPOA.[109] Such a link has previously been suggested and is particularly interesting in light of the role of prostaglandins in bone resorption and the observation that the genetic cause of the primary form of this condition also results in increased PGE-2.[110]

INVOLVEMENT OF JOINTS AND THE ASSOCIATED STRUCTURES
Direct Invasion by Tumor

Malignant involvement of joints may be direct, with synovium or other associated tissue as the primary site of malignant transformation, or indirect, with joint tissues or juxtaarticular regions serving as a site of metastatic disease. Primary synovial tumors are very rare, as are tumors of juxtaarticular structures.[102] However, primary tumors of bone, including chondrosarcoma, osteogenic sarcoma, or giant-cell tumors, as well as lymphoma, may grow in periarticular or articular tissue. Joint pain and swelling, frequently of insidious onset, are the usual clinical findings. These symptoms may result from direct involvement of joint tissue by tumor or from a synovial inflammatory reaction to adjacent tumor.[111] Two additional rare tumors can be mentioned in this context because although they are benign, they are proliferative, present similarly with joint swelling and stiffness, and can be mistaken for inflammatory arthritis. Pigmented villonodular synovitis (PVNS) is a synovial tumor in which massively proliferative synovial tissue is infiltrated with hemosiderin-laden macrophages.[112] This hemosiderin gives a characteristic appearance on magnetic resonance imaging, which is the preferred diagnostic imaging modality when this diagnosis is suspected. PVNS usually occurs in a diffuse form that affects an entire joint, by far most commonly the knee, but PVNS of the hip, shoulder, and ankle is described. This condition also occurs in a more limited form in which only a portion of the joint, or more commonly a portion of a tendon sheath, is involved. In this case, it can be confused with a giant-cell synovioma, also referred to as nodular tenosynovitis.[113]

Leukemic arthritis, in which leukemia cells infiltrate a joint space, synovium, or adjacent bone marrow, also frequently causes joint pain and sometimes synovitis.[114,115] Frequently, the site of infiltration is the bone marrow adjacent to a joint, resulting in a monoarticular or an oligoarticular periarthritis with pain near or around a joint, which may lead the patient and perhaps the unsuspecting physician to conclude it as arthritis. However, in these cases, bone pain can be more specifically localized by percussion of bone proximal to the joint and comparing the degree of tenderness elicited to that with joint palpation of movement. Benign osteoid tumors can produce similar symptoms.[102] Leukemic arthritis seems to occur more frequently in children than adults but does occur in both.[116–118]

Paraneoplastic Arthritis

Although direct joint involvement by cancer is unusual, several paraneoplastic syndromes include arthralgia and/or arthritis as part of their typical presentation. Inflammatory polyarthritis has been associated with many cancers. The onset of symptoms is frequently rapid, even explosive, but may also be more gradual. The presentation of inflammatory neoplastic arthropathy, sometimes called carcinoma polyarthritis, may be confused with rheumatoid arthritis (RA), particularly late-onset RA.[119] Late-onset RA is generally defined as the onset of disease after 60 years of age. Compared with typical RA, patients with late-onset disease are commonly seronegative for rheumatoid factor and cyclic citrullinated peptide (CCP) antibodies and are more commonly men.[120,121] It is particularly important to consider the possibility of cancer-associated polyarthritis in these patients because this is the same age group with increased cancer risk. However, compared with RA, the paraneoplastic presentation of polyarthritis is more likely to include other constitutional symptoms, including fever and markedly elevated acute-phase reactants. As a result, this condition may also be confused with other rheumatic diseases, including vasculitis and Still's disease.[119] Patients with cancer-related arthritis may also have other general signs of immune activation, including immune complex formation and production of antinuclear antibodies and rheumatoid factor.[122] However, the pathogenesis of the joint inflammation in this condition is unknown, and immune complex deposition is not reliably present in the joint tissue.[123] The most commonly reported underlying malignancies are solid tumors, particularly lung cancer and breast cancer in women.[124] The arthritis symptoms usually respond poorly to disease-modifying agents, and symptoms typically resolve with a successful tumor therapy.[124]

Remitting Seronegative Symmetric Synovitis with Pitting Edema

Remitting seronegative symmetric synovitis with pitting edema (RS3PE) is a distinct form of inflammatory polyarthropathy that has variably been considered as a subset of RA, including part of the spectrum of late-onset RA, or as a separate unique condition.[125] RS3PE was originally characterized as a condition with polyarthritis including symmetric synovitis of the hands and ankles, with prominent pitting edema in the extremities, elevated acute-phase reactants, and negative rheumatoid factor. The arthritis of RS3PE is not erosive and usually responds very well to low-dose corticosteroids or other mild treatments, and there is generally an excellent prognosis. However, this syndrome has also been described in association with a variety of cancers in several case reports.[126–128] Not only was there close temporal association between the onset of arthritis and the diagnosis of malignancy, but also in some cases, the signs and symptoms of rheumatic disease resolved with successful treatment of the underlying cancer. Thus, an RS3PE-like presentation should also be considered part of the spectrum of cancer-associated arthritis.

VASCULITIS
Polymyalgia Rheumatica

RS3PE and late-onset RA may also be confused with polymyalgia rheumatica (PMR).[129,130] Although PMR also generally occurs in people older than 50 years, it is characterized by debilitating arthralgias in the shoulder and hip girdle regions, a markedly elevated sedimentation rate, and variable headache.[130] However, a significant number of individuals with PMR have peripheral arthritis that includes the hands and wrist and that may include joint swelling.[131] Although there is debate in the literature as to whether the incidence of malignancy is increased among patients with PMR, the symptoms of occult malignancy can mimic PMR.[132] PMR itself is associated with temporal arteritis, a form of vasculitis characterized by granulomatous inflammation of small and medium cranial vessels with disruption of the elastic lamina and formation of giant cells.[133] Temporal or giant-cell arteritis is present in approximately 25% of patients with PMR, which has led some to consider PMR as part of the spectrum of giant-cell arteritis.[134,135] Epidemiologic studies have also suggested an association between temporal arteritis and cancer, but the long interval between the diagnosis of the 2 conditions in many of the patients included in these studies suggests a coincidence of common conditions rather than a causal relationship. Nevertheless, several individual case reports of closely associated temporal arteritis and newly diagnosed cancer, including lung, breast, and cervical cancer; multiple myeloma; and chronic myelogenous leukemia, suggest the possibility that this form of vasculitis may occasionally occur as a paraneoplastic process. In addition, these cases, as well as reports of cancer mistakenly diagnosed as temporal arteritis, emphasize that the PMR-like presentation of occult malignancy may also include features suggesting temporal arteritis.[136,137]

Cutaneous Vasculitis

The most common vasculitis associated with malignancy is inflammation of small vessels that most commonly presents as cutaneous leukocytoclastic vasculitis.[138,139] Hematologic malignancies have been the most commonly identified associates, but other solid tumors are also reported in association with leukocytoclastic vasculitis.[140,141] Analogous to other forms of leukocytoclastic vasculitis, the development of cutaneous inflammation is thought to be the result of circulating immune complexes containing tumor antigens deposited along the vascular walls, leading to complement activation and vascular inflammation. Although often abrupt in onset, about one-third of leukocytoclastic vasculitis cases can precede the clinical appearance of cancer by weeks to months.[141] The onset of leukocytoclastic vasculitis after 50 years of age is associated with a higher risk of concomitant malignancy.[141,142] Sweet syndrome is a recurrent neutrophilic dermatosis with pathologic features of cutaneous vasculitis that presents with coincident fever, leukocytosis, and sometimes arthralgias. This syndrome can also develop in response to drugs, infection, or as part of a spectrum of autoimmune disease and has also been associated with leukemia.[143,144]

Systemic Vasculitis

Concurrence of other forms of systemic vasculitis and cancer is reported sporadically in the literature, but these cases are distinctly uncommon.[145] However, many forms of systemic vasculitis have been reported, including polyarteritis nodosa (PAN), Henoch-Schönlein purpura, and eosinophilic granulomatous polyangiitis (Churg-Strauss).[146–151] Assignment of cause and effect in malignancy-associated vasculitis is complicated by reports of increased risk of cancer in patients with vasculitis, including Henoch-Schönlein purpura and the antineutrophil cytoplasmic antibody–associated vasculitides granulomatous polyangiitis (Wegener) and microscopic polyangiitis.[152,153] A retrospective review of patients with coincident vasculitis and cancer in whom both vasculitis and malignancy were diagnosed at the Cleveland Clinic over an 18-year period produced 69,000 patients diagnosed with cancer, 2800 with some form of vasculitis and 69 with both. However, only 12 patients received both diagnoses within 12 months of each other.[154] Seven of these cases had leukocytoclastic vasculitis, and the others included granulomatous angiitis, PAN, and temporal arteritis. That this experience was at a large tertiary care center and a vasculitis referral center means that this experience is likely at the high end of estimates for the frequency of malignancy-associated vasculitis and emphasizes that this association is uncommon. Nevertheless, this is consistent with other observations, suggesting that vasculitis can occasionally be part of a neoplastic process.

SUMMARY

Taken together, the wide range of rheumatic and musculoskeletal conditions that can appear in association with cancer emphasizes that rheumatic disease is a major component of the spectrum of paraneoplastic manifestations. Although the pathogenetic mechanisms by which neoplasia causes these manifestations are only partially understood in select cases, it appears that many result from immune-mediated effects stimulated by tumor antigens of endocrine factors produced by tumors. The broad overlap in signs and symptoms of occult malignancy and systemic rheumatic disease, as well as the occurrence of distinct localized and systemic musculoskeletal and rheumatic syndromes in the presence of cancer, emphasizes the importance of considering and investigating the possibility of occult malignancy in the evaluation of patients with these symptoms. This is particularly important in older patients, those with atypical rheumatic disease, and those who do not respond appropriately to conventional immunosuppressive therapy.

REFERENCES

1. Vial T, Descotes J. Immunosuppressive drugs and cancer. Toxicology 2003;185: 229–40.
2. Thompson AE, Rieder SW, Pope JE. Tumor necrosis factor therapy and the risk of serious infection and malignancy in patients with early rheumatoid arthritis: a meta-analysis of randomized controlled trials. Arthritis Rheum 2011;63: 1479–85.
3. Gutierrez-Dalmau A, Campistol JM. Immunosuppressive therapy and malignancy in organ transplant recipients: a systematic review. Drugs 2007;67:1167–98.
4. Shimada T, Mizutani S, Muto T, et al. Cloning and characterization of FGF23 as a causative factor of tumor-induced osteomalacia. Proc Natl Acad Sci U S A 2001;98:6500–5.
5. Carpenter TO. Oncogenic osteomalacia—a complex dance of factors. N Engl J Med 2003;348:1705–8.
6. Dalmau J, Tuzun E, Wu HY, et al. Paraneoplastic anti-N-methyl-D-aspartate receptor encephalitis associated with ovarian teratoma. Ann Neurol 2007;61: 25–36.

7. Luca N, Daengsuwan T, Dalmau J, et al. Anti-N-methyl-D-aspartate receptor encephalitis: a newly recognized inflammatory brain disease in children. Arthritis Rheum 2011;63:2516–22.

8. Cupps TR, Edgar LC, Thomas CA, et al. Multiple mechanisms of B cell immuno-regulation in man after administration of in vivo corticosteroids. J Immunol 1984; 132:170–5.

9. Poole S, Fenske NA. Cutaneous markers of internal malignancy. II. Paraneoplastic dermatoses and environmental carcinogens. J Am Acad Dermatol 1993;28: 147–64.

10. Poole S, Fenske NA. Cutaneous markers of internal malignancy. I. Malignant involvement of the skin and the genodermatoses. J Am Acad Dermatol 1993; 28:1–13.

11. Pfinsgraff J, Buckingham RB, Killian PJ, et al. Palmar fasciitis and arthritis with malignant neoplasms: a paraneoplastic syndrome. Semin Arthritis Rheum 1986;16:118–25.

12. Alexandroff AB, Hazleman BL, Matthewson M, et al. Woody hands. Lancet 2003; 361:1344.

13. Haroon M, Phelan M. A paraneoplastic case of palmar fasciitis and polyarthritis syndrome. Nat Clin Pract Rheumatol 2008;4:274–7.

14. Dinakar P, Hoke A. Paraneoplastic fasciitis-panniculitis syndrome: a neurological point of view. Nat Clin Pract Neurol 2009;5:113–7.

15. Medsger TA, Dixon JA, Garwood VF. Palmar fasciitis and polyarthritis associated with ovarian carcinoma. Ann Intern Med 1982;96:424–31.

16. Shiel WC Jr, Prete PE, Jason M, et al. Palmar fasciitis and arthritis with ovarian and non-ovarian carcinomas. New syndrome. Am J Med 1985;79:640–4.

17. Baron M. Palmar fasciitis, polyarthritis, and carcinoma. Ann Intern Med 1982; 97:616.

18. Martorell EA, Murray PM, Peterson JJ, et al. Palmar fasciitis and arthritis syndrome associated with metastatic ovarian carcinoma: a report of four cases. J Hand Surg Am 2004;29:654–60.

19. Yogarajah M, Soh J, Lord B, et al. Palmar fasciitis and polyarthritis syndrome: a sign of ovarian malignancy. J R Soc Med 2008;101:473–5.

20. Scheinfeld N. A review of the cutaneous paraneoplastic associations and meta-static presentations of ovarian carcinoma. Clin Exp Dermatol 2008;33:10–5.

21. Krishna K, Yacoub A, Hutchins LF, et al. Palmar fasciitis with polyarthritis syndrome in a patient with breast cancer. Clin Rheumatol 2011;30:569–72.

22. Kase H, Aoki Y, Sugaya S, et al. Palmar fasciitis and polyarthritis associated with squamous cell carcinoma of the cervix. Int J Gynecol Cancer 2000;10:507–9.

23. Clarke LL, Kennedy CT, Hollingworth P. Palmar fasciitis and polyarthritis syndrome associated with transitional cell carcinoma of the bladder. J Am Acad Dermatol 2011;64:1159–63.

24. Docquier C, Majois F, Mitine C. Palmar fasciitis and arthritis: association with endometrial adenocarcinoma. Clin Rheumatol 2002;21:63–5.

25. Roman S, Tebib J, Scoazec JY, et al. Palmar fasciitis and paraneoplastic poly-arthritis associated with hepatocellular carcinoma. Gastroenterol Clin Biol 2001; 25:203–4 [in French].

26. Enomoto M, Takemura H, Suzuki M, et al. Palmar fasciitis and polyarthritis asso-ciated with gastric carcinoma: complete resolution after total gastrectomy. Intern Med 2000;39:754–7.

27. Sheehy C, Ryan JG, Kelly M, et al. Palmar fasciitis and polyarthritis syndrome associated with non-small-cell lung carcinoma. Clin Rheumatol 2007;26:1951–3.

28. Naschitz JE, Yeshurun D, Zuckerman E, et al. Cancer-associated fasciitis panniculitis. Cancer 1994;73:231–5.

29. Chiari H. Uber die sogenannte fettnecrose. Prager Medizinishe Wochenschrift 1883;8:285–6.

30. Bohn S, Buchner S, Itin P. Erythema nodosum: 112 cases. Epidemiology, clinical aspects and histopathology. Schweiz Med Wochenschr 1997;127:1168–76 [in German].

31. Yeung CK, Au WY, Trendal-Smith N, et al. Panniculitis heralding blastic transformation of myelofibrosis. Br J Dermatol 2001;144:905–6.

32. Ido T, Kiyohara T, Sawai T, et al. Fasciitis-panniculitis syndrome and advanced gastric adenocarcinoma in association with antibodies to single-stranded DNA. Br J Dermatol 2006;155:640–1.

33. Shbeeb MI, Duffy J, Bjornsson J, et al. Subcutaneous fat necrosis and polyarthritis associated with pancreatic disease. Arthritis Rheum 1996;39:1922–5.

34. Durden FM, Variyam E, Chren MM. Fat necrosis with features of erythema nodosum in a patient with metastatic pancreatic carcinoma. Int J Dermatol 1996;35:39–41.

35. Mourad FH, Hannoush HM, Bahlawan M, et al. Panniculitis and arthritis as the presenting manifestation of chronic pancreatitis. J Clin Gastroenterol 2001;32: 259–61.

36. Preiss JC, Faiss S, Loddenkemper C, et al. Pancreatic panniculitis in an 88-year-old man with neuroendocrine carcinoma. Digestion 2002;66:193–6.

37. Sagi L, Amichai B, Barzilai A, et al. Pancreatic panniculitis and carcinoma of the pancreas. Clin Exp Dermatol 2009;34:e205–7.

38. Borowicz J, Morrison M, Hogan D, et al. Subcutaneous fat necrosis/panniculitis and polyarthritis associated with acinar cell carcinoma of the pancreas: a rare presentation of pancreatitis, panniculitis and polyarthritis syndrome. J Drugs Dermatol 2010;9:1145–50.

39. Vasdev V, Bhakuni D, Narayanan K, et al. Intramedullary fat necrosis, polyarthritis and panniculitis with pancreatic tumor: a case report. Int J Rheum Dis 2010; 13:e74–8.

40. Szymanski FJ, Bluefarb SM. Nodular fat necrosis and pancreatic diseases. Arch Dermatol 1961;83:224–9.

41. Hughes SH, Apisarnthanarax P, Mullins F. Subcutaneous fat necrosis associated with pancreatic disease. Arch Dermatol 1975;111:506–10.

42. van der Zee JA, van Hillegersberg R, Toonstra J, et al. Subcutaneous nodules pointing towards pancreatic disease: pancreatic panniculitis. Dig Surg 2004; 21:275–6.

43. Gahr N, Technau K, Ghanem N. Intraductal papillary mucinous adenoma of the pancreas presenting with lobular panniculitis. Eur Radiol 2006;16:1397–8.

44. Hamzaoui A, Gassab E, Kochteli I, et al. Erythema nodosum revealing parathyroid carcinoma. Eur Ann Otorhinolaryngol Head Neck Dis 2011. [Epub ahead of print].

45. Perez NB, Bernad B, Narvaez J, et al. Erythema nodosum and lung cancer. Joint Bone Spine 2006;73:336–7.

46. Glinkov S, Krasnaliev I, Atanassova M, et al. Hepatocellular carcinoma associated with paraneoplastic erythema nodosum and polyarthritis. J Hepatol 2003;39:656–7.

47. Robertson JC, Eeles GH. Syndrome associated with pancreatic acinar cell carcinoma. Br Med J 1970;2:708–9.

48. Virshup AM, Sliwinski AJ. Polyarthritis and subcutaneous nodules associated with carcinoma of the pancreas. Arthritis Rheum 1973;16:388–92.

49. Roumm AD, Medsger TA Jr. Cancer and systemic sclerosis. An epidemiologic study. Arthritis Rheum 1985;28:1336–40.
50. Abu-Shakra M, Guillemin F, Lee P. Cancer in systemic sclerosis. Arthritis Rheum 1993;36:460–4.
51. Rosenthal AK, McLaughlin JK, Gridley G, et al. Incidence of cancer among patients with systemic sclerosis. Cancer 1995;76:910–4.
52. Derk CT, Rasheed M, Artlett CM, et al. A cohort study of cancer incidence in systemic sclerosis. J Rheumatol 2006;33:1113–6.
53. Olesen AB, Svaerke C, Farkas DK, et al. Systemic sclerosis and the risk of cancer: a nationwide population-based cohort study. Br J Dermatol 2010;163:800–6.
54. Alexandrescu DT, Bhagwati NS, Wiernik PH. Chemotherapy-induced scleroderma: a pleiomorphic syndrome. Clin Exp Dermatol 2005;30:141–5.
55. Konishi Y, Sato H, Sato N, et al. Scleroderma-like cutaneous lesions induced by paclitaxel and carboplatin for ovarian carcinoma, not a single course of carboplatin, but re-induced and worsened by previously administratrd paclitaxel. J Obstet Gynaecol Res 2010;36:693–6.
56. Maehana T, Mizuno T, Muto M, et al. Scleroderma-like skin sclerosis induced by docetaxel chemotherapy for hormone refractory prostate cancer: a case report. Nihon Hinyokika Gakkai Zasshi 2010;101:726–9 [in Japanese].
57. Launay D, Le Berre R, Hatron PY, et al. Association between systemic sclerosis and breast cancer: eight new cases and review of the literature. Clin Rheumatol 2004;23:516–22.
58. Lu TY, Hill CL, Pontifex EK, et al. Breast cancer and systemic sclerosis: a clinical description of 21 patients in a population-based cohort study. Rheumatol Int 2008;28:895–9.
59. Peters-Golden M, Wise RA, Hochberg M, et al. Incidence of lung cancer in systemic sclerosis. J Rheumatol 1985;12:1136–9.
60. Orphanos G, Ardavanis A, Charalambous P, et al. Systemic sclerosis associated with rectal cancer. Case report and a brief review of the literature. In Vivo 2008; 22:825–9.
61. Shah AA, Rosen A, Hummers L, et al. Close temporal relationship between onset of cancer and scleroderma in patients with RNA polymerase I/III antibodies. Arthritis Rheum 2010;62:2787–95.
62. Airo P, Ceribelli A, Cavazzana I, et al. Malignancies in Italian patients with systemic sclerosis positive for anti-RNA polymerase III antibodies. J Rheumatol 2011;38:1329–34.
63. Poszepczynska-Guigne E, Viguier M, Chosidow O, et al. Paraneoplastic acral vascular syndrome: epidemiologic features, clinical manifestations, and disease sequelae. J Am Acad Dermatol 2002;47:47–52.
64. Kopterides P, Tsavaris N, Tzioufas A, et al. Digital gangrene and Raynaud's phenomenon as complications of lung adenocarcinoma. Lancet Oncol 2004; 5:549.
65. Lambova SN, Muller-Ladner U. Capillaroscopic pattern in systemic sclerosis— an association with dynamics of processes of angio- and vasculogenesis. Microvasc Res 2010;80:534–9.
66. Fam AG. Paraneoplastic rheumatic syndromes. Baillieres Best Pract Res Clin Rheumatol 2000;14:515–33.
67. Bardwick PA, Zvaifler NJ, Gill GN, et al. Plasma cell dyscrasia with polyneuropathy, organomegaly, endocrinopathy, M protein, and skin changes: the POEMS syndrome. Report on two cases and a review of the literature. Medicine (Baltimore) 1980;59:311–22.

68. Nakanishi T. Crow-Fukase syndrome. Nihon Naika Gakkai Zasshi 1985;74: 1205–9 [in Japanese].
69. Pavord SR, Murphy PT, Mitchell VE. POEMS syndrome and Waldenstrom's macroglobulinaemia. J Clin Pathol 1996;49:181–2.
70. Soubrier MJ, Dubost JJ, Sauvezie BJ. POEMS syndrome: a study of 25 cases and a review of the literature. French Study Group on POEMS Syndrome. Am J Med 1994;97:543–53.
71. Fishel B, Brenner S, Weiss S, et al. POEMS syndrome associated with cryoglobulinemia, lymphoma, multiple seborrheic keratosis, and ichthyosis. J Am Acad Dermatol 1988;19:979–82.
72. Watanabe O, Arimura K, Kitajima I, et al. Greatly raised vascular endothelial growth factor (VEGF) in POEMS syndrome. Lancet 1996;347:702.
73. Soubrier M, Dubost JJ, Serre AF, et al. Growth factors in POEMS syndrome: evidence for a marked increase in circulating vascular endothelial growth factor. Arthritis Rheum 1997;40:786–7.
74. Shibata M, Yamada T, Tanahashi N, et al. POEMS syndrome with necrotizing vasculitis: a novel feature of vascular abnormalities. Neurology 2000;54:772–3.
75. Badros A, Porter N, Zimrin A. Bevacizumab therapy for POEMS syndrome. Blood 2005;106:1135.
76. Samaras P, Bauer S, Stenner-Liewen F, et al. Treatment of POEMS syndrome with bevacizumab. Haematologica 2007;92:1438–9.
77. Kanai K, Kuwabara S, Misawa S, et al. Failure of treatment with anti-VEGF monoclonal antibody for long-standing POEMS syndrome. Intern Med 2007;46:311–3.
78. Dalakas MC, Hohlfeld R. Polymyositis and dermatomyositis. Lancet 2003;362: 971–82.
79. Sigurgeirsson B, Lindelof B, Edhag O, et al. Risk of cancer in patients with dermatomyositis or polymyositis. A population-based study. N Engl J Med 1992;326:363–7.
80. Zantos D, Zhang Y, Felson D. The overall and temporal association of cancer with polymyositis and dermatomyositis. J Rheumatol 1994;21:1855–9.
81. Callen JP. Myositis and malignancy. Curr Opin Rheumatol 1994;6:590–4.
82. Buchbinder R, Forbes A, Hall S, et al. Incidence of malignant disease in biopsy-proven inflammatory myopathy. A population-based cohort study. Ann Intern Med 2001;134:1087–95.
83. Hill CL, Zhang Y, Sigurgeirsson B, et al. Frequency of specific cancer types in dermatomyositis and polymyositis: a population-based study. Lancet 2001; 357:96–100.
84. Callen JP. When and how should the patient with dermatomyositis or amyopathic dermatomyositis be assessed for possible cancer? Arch Dermatol 2002;138:969–71.
85. Airio A, Pukkala E, Isomaki H. Elevated cancer incidence in patients with dermatomyositis: a population based study. J Rheumatol 1995;22:1300–3.
86. Stockton D, Doherty VR, Brewster DH. Risk of cancer in patients with dermatomyositis or polymyositis, and follow-up implications: a Scottish population-based cohort study. Br J Cancer 2001;85:41–5.
87. Alexandrescu DT, Bhagwati NS, Fomberstein B, et al. Steroid-responsive inclusion body myositis associated with endometrial cancer. Clin Exp Rheumatol 2005;23:93–6.
88. Euwer RL, Sontheimer RD. Amyopathic dermatomyositis (dermatomyositis sine myositis). Presentation of six new cases and review of the literature. J Am Acad Dermatol 1991;24:959–66.

89. Whitmore SE, Watson R, Rosenshein NB, et al. Dermatomyositis sine myositis: association with malignancy. J Rheumatol 1996;23:101–5.

90. Ebringer R, Rook G, Swana GT, et al. Autoantibodies to cartilage and type II collagen in relapsing polychondritis and other rheumatic diseases. Ann Rheum Dis 1981;40:473–9.

91. Buckner JH, Van Landeghen M, Kwok WW, et al. Identification of type II collagen peptide 261–273-specific T cell clones in a patient with relapsing polychondritis. Arthritis Rheum 2002;46:238–44.

92. Trentham DE, Le CH. Relapsing polychondritis. Ann Intern Med 1998;129: 114–22.

93. Hebbar M, Brouillard M, Wattel E, et al. Association of myelodysplastic syndrome and relapsing polychondritis: further evidence. Leukemia 1995;9:731–3.

94. Barzegar C, Vrtovsnik F, Devars JF, et al. Vasculitis with mesangial IgA deposits complicating relapsing polychondritis. Clin Exp Rheumatol 2002;20:89–91.

95. Cohen PR. Granuloma annulare, relapsing polychondritis, sarcoidosis, and systemic lupus erythematosus: conditions whose dermatologic manifestations may occur as hematologic malignancy-associated mucocutaneous paraneoplastic syndromes. Int J Dermatol 2006;45:70–80.

96. Yanagi T, Matsumura T, Kamekura R, et al. Relapsing polychondritis and malignant lymphoma: is polychondritis paraneoplastic? Arch Dermatol 2007;143: 89–90.

97. Martinez-Lavin M, Pineda C, Navarro C, et al. Primary hypertrophic osteoarthropathy: another heritable disorder associated with patent ductus arteriosus. Pediatr Cardiol 1993;14:181–2.

98. Schumacher HR Jr. Articular manifestations of hypertrophic pulmonary osteoarthropathy in bronchogenic carcinoma. Arthritis Rheum 1976;19:629–36.

99. Martinez-Lavin M, Matucci-Cerinic M, Jajic I, et al. Hypertrophic osteoarthropathy: consensus on its definition, classification, assessment and diagnostic criteria. J Rheumatol 1993;20:1386–7.

100. Uppal S, Diggle CP, Carr IM, et al. Mutations in 15-hydroxyprostaglandin dehydrogenase cause primary hypertrophic osteoarthropathy. Nat Genet 2008;40:789–93.

101. de Vernejoul MC, Kornak U. Heritable sclerosing bone disorders: presentation and new molecular mechanisms. Ann N Y Acad Sci 2010;1192:269–77.

102. Caldwell DS, McCallum RM. Rheumatologic manifestations of cancer. Med Clin North Am 1986;70:385–417.

103. Castori M, Sinibaldi L, Mingarelli R, et al. Pachydermoperiostosis: an update. Clin Genet 2005;68:477–86.

104. Martinez-Lavin M. Hypertrophic osteoarthropathy. Curr Opin Rheumatol 1997;9: 83–6.

105. Dickinson CJ, Martin JF. Megakaryocytes and platelet clumps as the cause of finger clubbing. Lancet 1987;2:1434–5.

106. Silveira LH, Martinez-Lavin M, Pineda C, et al. Vascular endothelial growth factor and hypertrophic osteoarthropathy. Clin Exp Rheumatol 2000;18:57–62.

107. Olan F, Portela M, Navarro C, et al. Circulating vascular endothelial growth factor concentrations in a case of pulmonary hypertrophic osteoarthropathy. Correlation with disease activity. J Rheumatol 2004;31:614–6.

108. Angel-Moreno Maroto A, Martinez-Quintana E, Suarez-Castellano L, et al. Painful hypertrophic osteoarthropathy successfully treated with octreotide. The pathogenetic role of vascular endothelial growth factor (VEGF). Rheumatology (Oxford) 2005;44:1326–7.

109. Kozak KR, Milne GL, Morrow JD, et al. Hypertrophic osteoarthropathy pathogenesis: a case highlighting the potential role for cyclo-oxygenase-2-derived prostaglandin E2. Nat Clin Pract Rheumatol 2006;2:452–6 [quiz: 456].

110. Norrdin RW, Jee WS, High WB. The role of prostaglandins in bone in vivo. Prostaglandins Leukot Essent Fatty Acids 1990;41:139–49.

111. Lagier R. Synovial reaction caused by adjacent malignant tumors: anatomicopathological study of three cases. J Rheumatol 1977;4:65–72.

112. Frassica FJ, Bhimani MA, McCarthy EF, et al. Pigmented villonodular synovitis of the hip and knee. Am Fam Physician 1999;60:1404–10 [discussion: 1415].

113. Jelinek JS, Kransdorf MJ, Shmookler BM, et al. Giant cell tumor of the tendon sheath: MR findings in nine cases. AJR Am J Roentgenol 1994;162:919–22.

114. Holdrinet RS, Corstens F, van Horn JR, et al. Leukemic synovitis. Am J Med 1989;86:123–6.

115. Evans TI, Nercessian BM, Sanders KM. Leukemic arthritis. Semin Arthritis Rheum 1994;24:48–56.

116. Fink CW, Windmiller J, Sartain P. Arthritis as the presenting feature of childhood leukemia. Arthritis Rheum 1972;15:347–9.

117. Bradlow A, Barton C. Arthritic presentation of childhood leukaemia. Postgrad Med J 1991;67:562–4.

118. Eguchi K, Aoyagi T, Nakashima M, et al. A case of adult T cell leukemia complicated by proliferative synovitis. J Rheumatol 1991;18:297–9.

119. Bennett RM, Ginsberg MH, Thomsen S. Carcinomatous polyarthritis. The presenting symptom of an ovarian tumor and association with a platelet activating factor. Arthritis Rheum 1976;19:953–8.

120. Turkcapar N, Demir O, Atli T, et al. Late onset rheumatoid arthritis: clinical and laboratory comparisons with younger onset patients. Arch Gerontol Geriatr 2006;42:225–31.

121. Olivieri I, Pipitone N, D'Angelo S, et al. Late-onset rheumatoid arthritis and late-onset spondyloarthritis. Clin Exp Rheumatol 2009;27:S139–45.

122. Marcus RM, Grayzel AI. A lupus antibody syndrome associated with hypernephroma. Arthritis Rheum 1979;22:1396–8.

123. Bradley JD, Pinals RS. Carcinoma polyarthritis: role of immune complexes in pathogenesis. J Rheumatol 1983;10:826–8.

124. Sheon RP, Kirsner AB, Tangsintanapas P, et al. Malignancy in rheumatic disease: interrelationships. J Am Geriatr Soc 1977;25:20–7.

125. McCarty DJ, O'Duffy JD, Pearson L, et al. Remitting seronegative symmetrical synovitis with pitting edema. RS3PE syndrome. JAMA 1985;254:2763–7.

126. Chiappetta N, Gruber B. Remitting seronegative symmetrical synovitis with pitting edema associated with acute myeloid leukemia. J Rheumatol 2005;32:1613–4.

127. Mattace-Raso FU, van der Cammen TJ. Remitting seronegative symmetrical synovitis with pitting oedema associated with lung malignancy. Age Ageing 2007;36:470–1.

128. Marto G, Klitna Z, Bileu MC, et al. Remitting seronegative symmetrical synovitis with pitting oedema syndrome, associated with prostate adenocarcinoma: a case report. Acta Reumatol Port 2010;35:358–60.

129. McCarty DJ. Comparison of polymyalgia rheumatica and remitting seronegative symmetrical synovitis with pitting edema syndrome: comment on the article by Salvarani et al. Arthritis Rheum 1996;39:1931–2.

130. Pease CT, Haugeberg G, Montague B, et al. Polymyalgia rheumatica can be distinguished from late onset rheumatoid arthritis at baseline: results of a 5-yr prospective study. Rheumatology (Oxford) 2009;48:123–7.

131. Salvarani C, Gabriel S, Hunder GG. Distal extremity swelling with pitting edema in polymyalgia rheumatica. Report on nineteen cases. Arthritis Rheum 1996;39: 73–80.

132. Naschitz JE, Slobodin G, Yeshurun D, et al. Atypical polymyalgia rheumatica as a presentation of metastatic cancer. Arch Intern Med 1997;157:2381.

133. Hunder GG. Giant cell arteritis and polymyalgia rheumatica. Med Clin North Am 1997;81:195–219.

134. Hunder GG. Giant cell arteritis in polymyalgia rheumatica. Am J Med 1997;102: 514–6.

135. Salvarani C, Cantini F, Boiardi L, et al. Polymyalgia rheumatica and giant-cell arteritis. N Engl J Med 2002;347:261–71.

136. Hammoudeh M, Khan MA. Cranial arteritis as the initial manifestation of malignant histiocytosis. J Rheumatol 1982;9:443–7.

137. Speed CA, Haslock I. Polymyalgia rheumatica, temporal arteritis and malignancy. Postgrad Med J 1995;71:500–2.

138. Mertz LE, Conn DL. Vasculitis associated with malignancy. Curr Opin Rheumatol 1992;4:39–46.

139. Garcia-Porrua C, Gonzalez-Gay MA. Cutaneous vasculitis as a paraneoplastic syndrome in adults. Arthritis Rheum 1998;41:1133–5.

140. Patel AM, Davila DG, Peters SG. Paraneoplastic syndromes associated with lung cancer. Mayo Clin Proc 1993;68:278–87.

141. Kurzrock R, Cohen PR. Cutaneous paraneoplastic syndromes in solid tumors. Am J Med 1995;99:662–71.

142. Sanchez-Guerrero J, Gutierrez-Urena S, Vidaller A, et al. Vasculitis as a paraneoplastic syndrome. Report of 11 cases and review of the literature. J Rheumatol 1990;17:1458–62.

143. Spector JI, Zimbler H, Levine R, et al. Sweet's syndrome. Association with acute leukemia. JAMA 1980;244:1131–2.

144. Cohen PR. Neutrophilic dermatoses occurring in oncology patients. Int J Dermatol 2007;46:106–11.

145. Greer JM, Longley S, Edwards NL, et al. Vasculitis associated with malignancy. Experience with 13 patients and literature review. Medicine (Baltimore) 1988;67: 220–30.

146. Gerber MA, Brodin A, Steinberg D, et al. Periarteritis nodosa, Australia antigen and lymphatic leukemia. N Engl J Med 1972;286:14–7.

147. Elkon KB, Hughes GR, Catovsky D, et al. Hairy-cell leukaemia with polyarteritis nodosa. Lancet 1979;2:280–2.

148. Cairns SA, Mallick NP, Lawler W, et al. Squamous cell carcinoma of bronchus presenting with Henoch-Schönlein purpura. Br Med J 1978;2:474–5.

149. Garcias VA, Herr HW. Henoch-Schönlein purpura associated with cancer of prostate. Urology 1982;19:155–8.

150. Vesole DH. Diffuse large-cell lymphoma in an adult with Schönlein-Henoch purpura. Arch Intern Med 1987;147:2026–7.

151. Cupps TR, Fauci AS. Neoplasm and systemic vasculitis: a case report. Arthritis Rheum 1982;25:475–6.

152. Pertuiset E, Liote F, Launay-Russ E, et al. Adult Henoch-Schönlein purpura associated with malignancy. Semin Arthritis Rheum 2000;29:360–7.

153. Pankhurst T, Savage CO, Gordon C, et al. Malignancy is increased in ANCA-associated vasculitis. Rheumatology (Oxford) 2004;43;1532–5.

154. Hutson TE, Hoffman GS. Temporal concurrence of vasculitis and cancer: a report of 12 cases. Arthritis Care Res 2000;13:417–23.

Serologic Laboratory Findings in Malignancy

Félix Fernández Madrid, MD, PhD*, Marie-Claire Maroun, MD

KEYWORDS

- Cancer • Autoantibodies • Autoimmunity
- Antinuclear antibodies • Antiphospholipid antibodies

Serologic findings such as antinuclear antibodies (ANA), usually found in systemic rheumatic diseases, have been known for decades to occur in patients with various cancers.[1,2] These and other early reports on ANAs in cancer sera[3–8] and the remarkable work responsible for the well-recognized value of autoantibodies for the diagnosis of autoimmune diseases (ADs) such as systemic lupus erythematosus (SLE), scleroderma, and dermatomyositis (DM)/polymyositis (PM)[9–13] suggested that autoantibodies could also be potential diagnostic and prognostic biomarkers for cancer. Biomarker discovery using genomics[14–21] and proteomics[22,23] led to the identification of a multitude of autoantibodies in various types of cancer, some of which appeared to be potential biomarkers for the diagnosis and prognosis of cancer.[16–21] Other approaches using antigens known to be involved in carcinogenesis showed that autoantibodies can also be used as potential diagnostic biomarkers.[24–26] However, ANAs in cancer sera were for a long time regarded as epiphenomena without any clinical significance. The interpretation of the significance of autoantibodies in cancer sera remained controversial, because although there are examples of autoantibodies commonly found in the ADs such as anti-DNA, anti-Sm, anti-RNP, and other antibodies,[27–31] a large number of the autoantibodies found in cancer sera do not recognize the autoantigens classically associated with the ADs.[15–17,22] These conflicting data were generally interpreted as an indication of the nonspecificity of autoantibodies in cancer sera. However, exceptions were known to occur, and a relatively small but steadily increasing group of autoantibodies recognizing the same antigens have been reported in both cancer and autoimmune sera. It is well known that patients with cancer may develop rheumatic, neurologic, and other symptoms generally thought to result from reactivity of autoantibodies with autoantigens located in tissues other than the primary tumor. The discussion of the clinical features as well as the serologic findings in cancer patients with paraneoplastic syndromes,[32–34] as well as those in

Part of this work was supported by R01 CA 122277 from the NCI.

The authors have nothing to disclose.

Division of Rheumatology, University Health Center, Wayne State University, 4201 Saint Antoine Pod 4H, Detroit, MI 48201, USA

* Corresponding author.

E-mail address: fmadrid@med.wayne.edu

Rheum Dis Clin N Am 37 (2011) 507–525

doi:10.1016/j.rdc.2011.09.006

0889-857X/11/$ – see front matter © 2011 Published by Elsevier Inc.

rheumatic.theclinics.com

cancer developing in patients with rheumatic diseases,[35–38] are outside of the scope of this review. Space limitations preclude the discussion of other important serologic findings in cancer sera, such as the cytokines, which have been covered in several publications.[39–41]

This review discusses serologic laboratory findings in malignancy of interest to rheumatologists as well as oncologists, from both the practical and basic viewpoints. Because of the potential significance of the use of autoantibodies for the screening and diagnosis of solid tumors, the article reviews primarily the work intending to identify diagnostic biomarkers for cancer and the number of autoantibodies common to the systemic ADs and cancer. Hundreds of autoantibodies recognizing tumor-associated antigens (TAAs) have been reported and reviewed in the past, and by necessity their discussion in this review is limited. The serologic findings in the sera of patients with solid tumors and hematological malignancies that the clinician may encounter in the practice of medicine are also reviewed. Finally, in view of the provocative recent data on the diagnostic and prognostic value of autoantibodies in cancer sera obtained using genomics and proteomics methodologies and the increasing recognition of an important role of B cells in the anticancer immune response,[42–47] the potential significance of the prominent autoantibody response in cancer sera is discussed.

AUTOANTIBODIES AS POTENTIAL DIAGNOSTIC BIOMARKERS OF SOLID TUMORS

Cancer sera contain antibodies that react with a unique group of autologous cellular antigens called TAAs. Many studies have demonstrated that single antibody specificities recognize their corresponding autoantigens in a range from 10% to 20%, which is not satisfactory for diagnostic purposes, and there is general agreement that panels of autoantibodies are superior to single autoantibody markers as potential diagnostic markers in cancer.[15,16,18–21,24,48,49] Autoantibody panels with relatively high sensitivity and specificity have been reported for several cancers.[16,18–21] However, the levels of sensitivity and specificity achieved thus far do not seem sufficiently high to be useful in the clinical arena. Further work will be necessary to improve the accuracy of autoantibody panels to levels that could be helpful for the clinician. This task is a challenging one that will involve the refining of the reported diagnostic panels, and should culminate in the prospective validation of such panels with independent collections sera from cancer patients and controls. Validation is a prerequisite for any diagnostic autoantibody panel before its use in the clinical laboratory and its introduction in clinical trials. Problems encountered by these studies include the selection and recruiting of large numbers of cancer patients and controls required to achieve statistical significance. Multiple studies have found that potential TAAs manifest reactivity with sera from control donors. On this basis, the validation of antigen-antibody systems with cancer-related serologic profile is a complex task requiring a large number of sera from cases and controls. Not only should the numbers of control sera be sufficient for statistical evaluation of the data on autoantibody reactivity, but the choice of controls is of utmost importance. The use of control subjects drawn from the population at risk for a given cancer is probably the preferred method, because data showing statistical significance obtained using convenience controls may not stand using real-life controls. Many studies have used high-throughput microarray or proteomics platforms that are labor intensive and very complex, and although highly adequate for biomarker discovery, these are not suitable for use at the clinical laboratory level. Thus, once a diagnostic instrument based on autoantibodies has achieved sufficiently high accuracy to identify cases and controls at the biodiscovery level, other more flexible and easy-to-use platforms such as specific enzyme-linked immunosorbent assays (ELISAs), or other platforms based on bioluminescence, will probably be used to test the diagnostic panels in clinical studies. There is presently a great deal of interest in these studies that promise to promote the early diagnosis of cancer.

Several different approaches have been used thus far for biomarker discovery. Some studies were based on the construction of microarrays using collections of proteins known to be involved in carcinogenesis, which are recognized as autoantigens in various malignancies.[24,48,49] These microcollections are hybridized with sera from cancer patients and controls using high-throughput autoantigen microarray technology or ELISA platforms. Using this approach, Zhang and colleagues[24] reported that a mini-array of multiple TAAs would enhance antibody detection and could be a useful approach for cancer detection. These investigators used full-length recombinant proteins expressed from cDNAs encoding c-myc, p53, cyclin B1, p62, Koc, IMP1, and survivin in a diagnostic mini-array. Enzyme immunoassay was used to detect antibodies in sera from 6 different types of cancers. Antibody frequency to any individual TAA was variable but rarely exceeded 15% to 20%. With the successive addition of TAAs to a total of 7 antigens, there was a stepwise increase of positive antibody reactions up to a range of 44% to 68%, showing the advantages of using a panel of TAAs rather than single specificities. Sera from patients with breast, lung, and prostate cancer showed separate and distinct profiles of reactivity, suggesting that uniquely constituted antigen mini-arrays might be developed to distinguish between some types of cancer. It was proposed that detection of autoantibodies in cancer sera can be enhanced by using a mini-array of several TAAs as target antigens. Chapman and colleagues[48] used a quality-controlled, semi-automated indirect ELISA to test a panel of 7 antigens comprising several well-recognized cancer-associated proteins including the c-myc oncogene, p53, HER2, MUC1, NY-ESO-1, CAGE, and GBU4-5. These proteins were selected because they are known to be involved in the carcinogenic process, to be aberrantly expressed on the cell surface of solid tumors, or to induce autoantibody responses in cancer sera. One of these antigens, GBU4-5 encoding a DEAD box domain, is of interest because DEAD box–containing proteins are involved in RNA processing, ribosome assembly, spermatogenesis, embryogenesis, and cell growth and division. Using this approach Chapman's group reported elevated levels of autoantibodies to at least 1 of the 7 antigens in the panel, in 76% of lung cancer (LC) patients tested, with a specificity of 92%. There was no significant difference between the detection rates in the LC subgroups. More recently, this group confirmed the value of an autoantibody panel as a diagnostic tool in 3 cohorts of patients with newly diagnosed LC, and potentially able to identify patients at high risk of LC. Autoantibody levels were measured against a panel constructed with p53, NY-ESO-1, CAGE, GBU4-5, annexin 1, and SOX2. This panel demonstrated a sensitivity/specificity of 36%/91%, 39%/89%, and 37%/90% in the 3 cohorts of LC patients with good reproducibility. The advantages of this approach are that the proteins tested in the mini-arrays are known to be involved in important aspects of carcinogenesis, that the antigens printed are recombinant proteins, and that the platforms used could be more easily adapted for cancer detection in the clinical laboratories. The disadvantages of this approach are that the choice of antigens is arbitrary and that the antigens tested are common to several cancers and not necessarily specific for the tumor of interest. This objection is not a serious one, because reactivities shared by several cancers may contribute to a diagnostic panel showing high specificity for the tumor. The expectation using this approach is that the addition of new antigens will be able to produce a diagnostic panel with sufficiently high accuracy to be useful in the clinical arena.

Other investigators have attempted to identify TAAs recognized by serum antibodies using proteomics[22,23] or genomics[14,15] methodologies. The use of proteomics has led to the identification of a large group of autoantigens recognized by cancer sera. An example of this approach is the report of Brichory and colleagues,[50] who implemented a proteomics approach for the identification of tumor antigens that elicit a humoral response. These investigators used 2-dimensional polyacrylamide gel electrophoresis to simultaneously separate several thousand individual cellular proteins from tumor tissue or tumor cell lines. Separated proteins were transferred onto membranes, and sera from cancer patients were screened individually by Western blot analysis for antibodies that react against separated proteins. Proteins that specifically reacted with sera from cancer patients were identified by mass spectrometric analysis. The investigators reported the identification of autoantibodies reacting against a group of 4 25-kDa proteins identified as PGP 9.5 in 9 of 64 sera. Their findings suggested that ectopic expression of PGP 9.5 and release into the serum are associated with a humoral response detectable in a subset of LC patients.

The genomic approach uses immunoscreening cDNA libraries constructed from mRNA isolated from tumor tissues or from established cancer cell lines to identify TAAs targeted by autoantibodies.[14–21] Immunoscreening expression libraries has been used for several decades, and since the report of Carlsson and colleagues,[51] some changes in the original procedure have been introduced. Immunoscreening cDNA expression libraries using SEREX (Serologic analysis of cDNA expression libraries)[14] resulted in the identification of a broad spectrum of candidate tumor antigens.[14,15] SEREX analysis involves immunoscreening of expression libraries with autologous patients' serum, identification of gene products encoded by positive clones, analysis of mRNA expression, and evaluation of the seroreactivity of autoantigen panels using sera from cases and controls. Two main strategies commonly used for the determination of serologic profiles of antigens identified by biopanning cDNA libraries are a small-scale conventional serologic survey, also called petit serology, and an ELISA using purified recombinant proteins as substrate.[15] Petit serology directly uses crude phage lysates and requires large volumes of sera individually preadsorbed with *Escherichia coli* phage lysates. The disadvantages of petit serology are that large volumes of sera from large numbers of patients and controls are difficult to obtain, the procedure is labor intensive, and it does not easily lend itself to high throughput. Determination of serum autoreactivity by ELISA requires purified recombinant proteins as substrate. The system is more simple and manageable because the substrate is devoid of phage particles and can be quite robust. Moreover, ELISA could be more easily adapted for use in clinical trials than autoantigen microarrays. Subsequently, many studies used array-based methods using different formats and detection principles.[52–58] Lagarkova and colleagues[58] described SMARTA (serologic mini-arrays of recombinant tumor antigens), an improved version of allogeneic screening protocol for testing SEREX-defined recombinant clones using serologic mini-arrays in 96-well format. This method was thought to be useful for extensive serologic analysis of a small panel of preselected recombinant antigens, providing a desirable balance between labor-intensive conventional screening as proposed by classic SEREX and expensive robot-assisted autoantigen microarray analysis.[58] Modifications of the immunoscreening procedure used to identify the potential TAAs have been proposed,[16,59] including the use of cDNA libraries prepared with mRNA from heterologous cancer donors, and the selection of cloning sera containing high-titer IgG antibodies. These and other modifications intend to allow the identification of autoantigens relevant to the process of carcinogenesis, which could contribute to a diagnostic panel with high sensitivity and specificity useful in the clinical setting.

Using autoantigen microarray methodology, the amplified colonies identified by immunoscreening are printed as a microarray on treated glass slides and hybridized with sera from cancer patients and controls. Following this procedure, the authors have reported a 12-phage breast cancer predictor group constructed with phage inserts recognized by sera from patients with breast cancer and not by noncancer or autoimmune control sera. Several autoantigens including annexin XI-A, the p80 subunit of the Ku antigen, ribosomal protein S6, and other unknown autoantigens were found to significantly discriminate between breast cancer and noncancer control sera. In addition, sequences identical to annexin XI-A, nucleolar protein interacting with the FHA domain of pKi-67, the KIAA1671 gene product, ribosomal protein S6, elongation factor-2, Grb2-associated protein 2, and other unknown proteins could distinguish ductal carcinoma in situ from invasive ductal carcinoma of the breast, and appear to be potential biomarkers for the diagnosis of breast cancer.[16,17] In further work, biopanning a T7 cDNA library of breast cancer proteins with breast cancer sera identified a small group of expression sequence tags with identity to the oncogene Bmi-1 and other proteins, having in common their ability to participate in regulatory processes such as self renewal and epigenetic chromatin remodeling.[60]

In aggregate, the serologic markers for the diagnosis of cancer reported thus far with antibody-based methods, though promising to revolutionize the fields of screening and early diagnosis of cancer, have not been definitively validated and exhibit limited specificity and sensitivity, insufficient for diagnostic or prognostic purposes in the clinical arena. Thus there is an urgent need to develop and, more importantly, to validate biomarkers with higher accuracy, which alone or in combination with other available screening methods, such as mammography in breast cancer[61] or low-dose helical computed tomography in LC,[62] might significantly improve the likelihood of detecting cancer at an earlier stage.

AUTOANTIBODIES COMMON TO AUTOIMMUNE DISEASES AND MALIGNANCIES FOUND IN CLINICAL PRACTICE
Antinuclear Antibodies

Antinuclear antibodies in malignancies have been reported for decades,[1,2] and this subject has been reviewed in the past.[35,63,64] Forty years ago, it was first suggested that the prevalence of ANAs is increased in patients with malignancies, particularly in breast cancer.[65] Subsequently, multiple case reports confirmed that ANAs are commonly found in sera of cancer patients,[1,2] and many studies involving large numbers of cancer-patient sera and noncancer controls have shown that ANAs are frequently identified in the sera of patients with neoplasms.[66–68] Immunofluorescence using HEp-2 cells became the gold standard for ANA determination in the clinical laboratory, and multiple techniques to detect ANAs have evolved during these 4 decades.[69–73]

In the practice of medicine, positive ANA tests are frequently reported in the general population, and their interpretation is often perplexing because no apparent cause of this finding is evident when the patient does not have a systemic AD. It has been thought for a long time that the frequency of autoantibodies increases with age. However, in the study of Li and colleagues,[74] age was not related to ANA positivity in healthy subjects who were negative for current or past ADs. It has been suggested that humans, as a species, may be predisposed to autoimmunity.[75] The influence of sex has been noted, because several works reported that ANA-positive tests are significantly more frequent in healthy females than in healthy males.[76,77] In this context, women are known to be more susceptible to some ADs such as SLE, rheumatoid arthritis (RA), Hashimoto thyroiditis, and primary biliary cirrhosis. This propensity of females to develop autoimmune processes has been also found in animal models of ADs.[78] It is not surprising that ANA test positivity is more frequent in females than in males, because it has been reported that women develop more robust immune responses than men.[79,80] The hormonal basis for sex differences in ADs that make women more at risk for a variety of ADs may also be pertinent to the pathogenesis of some solid tumors such as breast cancer. It has been reported that autoantibodies are typically present many years before the diagnosis of SLE (unpublished data), and the authors have made similar observations in patients with scleroderma and Hashimoto thyroiditis.[81] Relevant to the interpretation of a positive ANA test in a healthy person are the reports that autoantibodies can be detected in cancer sera many years before the clinical diagnosis of cancer.[5,82,83] Similarly, an unknown number of subjects who are at risk for neoplasia and will eventually develop cancer may have positive ANA tests, contributing also to the tip of the autoimmunity iceberg.[75] The implication of these findings is that many healthy subjects in the general population, who will eventually develop systemic ADs or cancer, may present positive serology for ANAs. In a survey of ANAs in a rheumatology practice, Shiel and colleagues[84] reported that in 2.9% of all patients with ANAs and no established diagnosis referred to a rheumatologist for evaluation, a neoplasia was found. The authors speculate that an unknown proportion of healthy persons who have the predisposition to develop an AD but never reach the clinical diagnostic threshold, and others who have premalignant changes but will or will not develop cancer, may also present with autoantibodies of unknown cause. It has been reported that up to 20% or more of otherwise healthy people can express ANAs. This interesting subject has been recently discussed.[74,75]

An increasing number of autoantibody specificities have been reported in the sera from cancer patients.[15–17,24,27–31,49] Imai and colleagues reported that patients with hepatocellular carcinoma (HCC), or gastrointestinal, lung, and ovarian cancers had autoantibodies to nuclear and nucleolar antigens detected by immunofluorescence on cell substrates. The frequency of ANAs was significantly higher in patients with HCC than in patients with chronic hepatitis or liver cirrhosis. A higher percentage of nucleolar fluorescence was detected in sera from patients with HCC, and 3 of these nucleolar antigens were identified as NOR-90, nucleolus organizer region doublet polypeptides of 93 and 89 kDa involved in RNA polymerase I transcription; fibrillarin, a 34-kDa protein of the nucleolar U3 ribonucleoprotein particle that is engaged in pre-ribosomal RNA processing; and nucleophosmin/protein B23, a 37 kDa polypeptide that is associated with ribosome maturation and cellular proliferation. These antigens are nucleolar components that are engaged in some aspect of ribosome biosynthesis. Autoantibodies to these nucleolar antigens have also been found in systemic ADs, and they do not represent autoimmune reactions unique to cancer. The investigators suggested that these antibodies might reflect reaction pathways related to immune responses that are antigen driven.[67] The report of Imai and colleagues is a classic example of the potential of autoantibodies to contribute significantly to patient care. In some patients with liver cirrhosis who developed HCC they observed seroconversion to ANA positivity, and a marked increase in titer and/or a change in antibody specificity preceding or coincident with clinical detection of HCC. These changes in ANA titer and/or specificity showed a close temporal relationship with transformation from long-established chronic liver disease to HCC.

Shoenfeld and colleagues[27,28] reported anti-DNA antibodies, anti-histone, and anti-Sm-RNP in the sera of patients with monoclonal gammopathies.[29] Anti-dsDNA autoantibodies were also reported in patients with colorectal adenocarcinoma.[30] Despite these isolated reports, in aggregate the literature on autoantibodies in cancer has not consistently demonstrated the ANA specificities characteristic of the systemic ADs such as SLE, scleroderma, or DM in cancer sera. This finding may simply reflect molecular differences between the autoantigens involved in cancer and those characteristically involved in the systemic ADs.

Antiphospholipid Antibodies

There is growing evidence on the association of antiphospholipid antibodies (aPL) with malignancies.[85] The antiphospholipid syndrome (APS) is a systemic autoimmune disorder characterized by a combination of arterial and/or venous thrombosis, recurrent fetal loss, often accompanied by a mild to moderate thrombocytopenia, and elevated titers of aPL.[86] aPL are directed predominantly against self protein phospholipid complexes. aPL reported in cancer sera include lupus anticoagulant (LAC), anticardiolipin antibodies (ACL), and α2-glycoprotein I. Conflicting results have been published on the association of aPL and the prevalence of thrombotic events. The prevalence of aPL in cancer sera is variable. In the report of Zuckerman and colleagues,[87] 22% of cancer sera were ACL positive compared with 3% of healthy controls. Patients with ACL-positive sera, mainly those with high titers, had a significantly higher rate of thromboembolic events than ACL-negative cancer patients. Of interest, the levels of aCL decreased 3 months after the initiation of successful treatment of cancer and remained negative during a 12-month follow-up period.[87] LAC was reported in 58% of patients with lung adenocarcinoma, and the investigators found a strong association of thrombosis with LAC but not with ACL in cancer patients.[88] Other studies demonstrated an increased prevalence of aPL in various malignancies, without increase of the risk for thrombosis.[89,90]

Lossos and colleagues[91] found ACLs in 68% of sera from patients with acute myeloid leukemia (AML) and an increase in their titers during AML relapses. However, the presence of ACL was not associated with an increased risk of thromboembolism. The investigators suggested that ACL could be a useful marker to assess relapses and disease activity.

Font and colleagues reported that the prevalence of aPL was higher in cancer patients with venous thromboembolism (VTE) than in patients without VTE and healthy subjects. The aPL positivity persisted in only 4 out of 21 patients, suggesting that aPL may not be pathogenic in the development of VTE observed in patients with solid malignancies.[92]

APS can be associated with ADs or with chronic infections,[93,94] and it has been observed that in these patients the aPL titers wax and wane throughout the course of the disease, but usually fail to disappear. However, when APS is associated with hematological malignancies, aPL have been shown to disappear after proper treatment.[85] Because diminishing the antigenic load may influence the aPL levels, this suggests that the antibody response might be triggered by tumor antigens.[87]

OTHER AUTOANTIBODIES COMMON TO CANCER AND AUTOIMMUNE RHEUMATIC DISEASES

There have been multiple reports of autoantibodies common to cancer and autoimmune rheumatic diseases which have been reviewed.[63,64] Here, the authors discuss only a few examples of this interesting association. p53 autoantibodies in cancer sera have been known to occur for 3 decades.[95] Crawford and colleagues described antibodies against human p53 in 9% of sera from breast cancer patients. Later, Caron de Fromentel and colleagues[96] found that anti-p53 antibodies were present in sera of children with cancer, in 21% with B-cell lymphomas, and in 12% with a wide range of tumor types. These studies remained largely unnoticed until the discovery in the early 1990s that the P53 gene is the most common target for molecular alteration in almost every type of human cancer, and subsequently the occurrence of p53 antibodies in cancer sera was confirmed, suggesting the possible value of p53 and other autoantibodies for the diagnosis of cancer. This subject has been comprehensively reviewed.[97] These autoantibodies do not have diagnostic specificity because they have been found in patients with various cancer types including lung, pancreas, bladder, breast, and ovarian cancers.[97] p53 is a nuclear transcription factor playing an important role in the control of cell proliferation and apoptosis. The p53 tumor suppressor protein arrests the cell cycle primarily at the G1 phase or induces apoptosis in response to cellular DNA damage, thus allowing DNA repair.[98] For these and other reasons, p53 has been called the "guardian of the genome."[99] The molecular process leading to the generation of p53 antibodies, in particular their association with mutations, has been studied in more detail than for any other antigen/antibody system in cancer sera.[100] These antibodies seem to result from the strong immunogenicity of the p53 protein, and although they may be associated with P53 gene missense mutations, p53 antibodies may react with epitopes in the wild-type protein. Those antibodies developing in patients with P53 mutations react with immunodominant epitopes and not necessarily with epitopes in the mutated part of the molecule.[100] Moreover, some patients with tumors having P53 mutations and expressing high levels of the mutant protein may not develop p53 antibodies. Autoantibodies against p53 have been detected in the sera of patients with several ADs including type 1 diabetes, thyroid disease, SLE, systemic sclerosis, overlap syndromes, and other rheumatic diseases.[101–104] The clinical value of anti-p53 antibodies in malignancies remains a subject of debate, but consistent results have been reported in breast, colon, head and neck, and gastric cancers, in which p53 antibodies have been associated with high-grade tumors and poor survival.[97,105–108] These reports suggest a potential prognostic value for p53 autoantibodies. The involvement of p53 in early stages of carcinogenesis is suggested by the finding of p53 antibodies months to years before the clinical diagnosis of cancer.[63,109] In agreement with this possibility, anti-p53 antibodies were found in the sera of workers exposed to vinyl chloride who later developed angiosarcoma of the liver, and in the sera of heavy smokers who eventually developed LC.[99] All these findings suggest that anti-p53 and other autoantibodies are potential biomarkers for the early detection of cancer. In breast cancer, it has been possible to detect the reappearance of these antibodies 3 months before the detection of a relapse. These autoantibodies are of the IgG class, indicating a secondary response after a prolonged immunization before the diagnosis of the disease.[97] Based on these studies, the authors speculate that autoantibodies may in the future be found to be helpful in the identification of healthy subjects at high risk for cancer, bearing premalignant changes.

Autoantibodies to c-myc have been reported in sera from patients with cancer and with ADs such as SLE, scleroderma, and DM.[100–112] The c-myc protein is a phosphorylated nuclear protein closely associated with the nuclear matrix.[113] Autoantibodies to c-myc have been reported in sera from patients with breast[111] and colorectal cancers,[113] and full-length recombinant c-myc tested in a mini-array has been shown to contribute to the sensitivity and specificity of a diagnostic autoantigen panel.[49]

Anti-Ku antibodies have been reported in cancer and autoimmune sera from patients with the scleroderma-polymyositis overlap syndrome.[114] DM and PM are inflammatory disorders characterized by muscle inflammation and a tendency to develop internal malignancy.[115] Autoimmunity is thought to play a critical role, and several characteristic autoantibodies have been described.[116,117] It is clear that the availability of biomarkers predicting the development of neoplasia in these patients would be very helpful for the clinician. Anti-Ku antibodies have been further reported in a small number of patients with several systemic ADs including SLE, scleroderma, and RA.[118] The heterodimeric Ku protein, composed of 86-kDa (Ku80) and 70-kDa (Ku70) subunits, is the DNA-targeting component of DNA-dependent protein kinase, which plays a critical role in mammalian DNA double-strand break repair[119] through the nonhomologous end-joining pathway.[120] The authors have reported antibodies to the p80 subunit of Ku antigen in sera of breast cancer patients.[16,17] The heterodimeric Ku protein has been widely implicated in tumor biology.[121] The finding of an autoimmune reaction directed toward the Ku antigen in the sera of cancer patients suggests that the molecular changes leading to autoimmunity of proteins involved in DNA repair may be important in breast carcinogenesis.

Anticollagen antibodies are common findings in the sera from patients with RA, SLE, relapsing polychondritis, and other autoimmune connective tissue disorders.[121–123] The authors' laboratory reported that autoimmunity to collagen antigens occurs frequently in patients with LC before initiation of therapy.[3–8] The prevalence of anticollagen antibodies was found to vary between 12% and 28% depending on the type of collagen, and overall, 43% of LC sera were positive for one or more collagen antigens. Subsequently the authors have found anticollagen antibodies with specificity for type I α2 chain in the sera of patients with breast cancer [unpublished data]. In the light of the recognized role of stromal proteins in the development and progression of cancer,[124,125] the authors speculate that anticollagen antibodies in cancer sera may reflect an autoimmune response to collagen macromolecules in the tumor stroma. Because autoantibodies to collagen macromolecules have been reported in the sera from patients with RA and SLE, the finding of anticollagen antibodies in lung and breast cancers and probably in other solid tumors is reminiscent of the findings in the systemic ADs.

Antibodies to annexin XI-A,[126] RPA32,[127] and elongation factor-2[128,129] have been reported in cancer sera[5,16,17] and autoimmune sera.[130–133] Annexin XI is a member of the annexin superfamily of Ca^{2+} and phospholipid-binding, membrane-associated proteins implicated in Ca^{2+}-signal transduction processes associated with cell growth and differentiation. Annexin XI may have a role in cellular DNA synthesis and in cell proliferation as well as in membrane trafficking events such as exocytosis, and has been found to be identical to a 56-kDa antigen recognized by antibodies in 3.9% of patients with systemic ADs.[130,131] The authors' laboratory has reported antiannexin XI-A antibodies in 19% of women with breast cancer and in 60% of sera from women with ductal carcinoma in situ of the breast.[16] The authors have also reported a prevalence of anti-RPA32 in 11% of breast cancer sera.[5] A parallel was found between breast cancer and ADs in reference to serum reactivity to annexin XI-A and RPA32, because the frequency of these antibodies in breast cancer sera (11%–19%) is substantially higher than in the systemic ADs such as SLE and Sjögren syndrome, which has been estimated to be 2% to 3% and 3.9%, respectively. It is pertinent that both SLE and Sjögren syndrome are known to be associated with a tendency to develop lymphoid malignancies.[134,135] There are reports on the cancer-predicting ability of several members of the large annexin family that are suspected to be involved in the process of carcinogenesis.[136–138] The authors have also reported that elongation factor 2 (EF-2) is recognized as an autoantigens by breast cancer sera.[16,17] EF-2 is phosphorylated by a calmodulin-dependent protein kinase, CaM K III, which is selectively activated in proliferating cells.[139] Of interest, Alberdi and colleagues[133] reported a cross-reaction between anti-dsDNA antibodies from patients with SLE and

EF-2, and demonstrated in vitro that this interaction could lead to cellular dysfunction, as evidenced by inhibition of protein synthesis, suggesting a direct pathogenic role for cell penetrating anti-dsDNA antibodies. Therefore, it is possible that the antibodies to RPA32, annexin XI-A, and EF-2 and other as yet unknown autoantigens in the sera of a small proportion of patients with systemic ADs may represent early markers of malignancy. The possibility of these autoantibodies being useful markers to identify patients with rheumatic diseases at risk of developing cancer could be investigated in prospective studies.

SIGNIFICANCE OF AUTOANTIBODIES IN CANCER SERA

The development of autoantibodies is the consequence of breakdown of immunologic tolerance, but their presence is not exclusive of autoimmune conditions.[63] Autoantibodies have been for years considered to be epiphenomena probably related to the breakdown and release of tumor proteins. Although the interpretation of positive serologic findings in cancer sera remains controversial, the significance of the autoantibodies observed in cancer can be viewed through the prism of the humoral autoimmune response in the autoimmune diseases.[7-9] Indeed, many of the features characterizing the autoantibody response in the ADs are mimicked by the humoral response in cancer sera. Although mutated proteins can elicit an autoantibody response and mutations are a prominent feature in carcinogenesis, the majority of the TAAs recognized by antibodies in cancer sera are abnormally expressed wild-type proteins and not the products of mutated genes. Several longitudinal cohort studies have shown that patients with ADs may develop autoantibodies many years before they manifest clinical symptoms.[81] Similarly, autoantibodies in cancer sera many appear many years before the diagnosis of cancer,[5,82,83] suggesting that the process leading to autoantibody formation in patients with cancer occurs during the very early stages of tumorigenesis. Frenkel and colleagues analyzed the sera of 169 women who were healthy at the time of blood donation for the presence of antibodies to 5-hydroxymethyl-2'-deoxyuridine, an oxidized DNA base, using ELISA. Sera collected 6 to 72 months before these women were discovered to have breast cancer showed significantly elevated levels of this antibody. The investigators suggested that this autoantibody potentially can serve as a marker for increased risk of breast cancer, because relatively high serum levels were also detected in otherwise healthy women with a first-degree family history of breast cancer and in women with the diagnosis of benign conditions.[83] Many of the cellular proteins recognized as autoantigens by serum antibodies are involved, as suggested by Tan,[9] in fundamental cellular functions such as DNA replication and transcription. This association has been confirmed in many studies.[7-9,15,17] The mechanisms that trigger humoral autoreactivity in cancer patients is complex and not completely understood, but seems to be the consequence of abnormal self-antigen expression by tumor cells and of the development of an inflammatory reaction within the tumor microenvironment.[31,140,141] Many recent studies on the significance of infiltrating lymphocytes in tumor tissue have provided evidence that B-cell autoreactivity is extremely important in cancer,[42-47] and together with the plethora of autoantibody specificities cloned by immunoscreening cDNA expression libraries[14-19,24,48,49] or by proteomics[22] found to be associated with cancer, suggest an antigen-driven humoral immune response. In agreement with this possibility, there is evidence that the majority of the autoantibodies detected in cancer sera found to be associated with diagnosis of the neoplasia are of the IgG class of immunoglobulins.[15-17]

As has been demonstrated in the systemic ADs, autoantibodies in cancer sera may have diagnostic and prognostic value and have the potential to detect cancer early, when the treatment has the best chance to affect tumor behavior. In support of this possibility, immunopathologic studies of premalignant disease have shown molecular alterations that have been associated with autoreactivity to cancer-associated proteins.[142]

The cancer stem cell hypothesis[143–145] may be relevant to the interpretation of auto-antibody tests in cancer sera. This hypothesis would have important implications for biomarker discovery, because it suggests that a small subset of tumor-initiating cells or stem cells is responsible for cancer initiation and recurrences. Malignant tumors are heterogeneous and antigen diverse, and an undetermined portion of the TAAs identified by autoantibodies, although indeed tumor associated, have probably originated in the bulk of the nontumorigenic but as yet antigenic cells. It is likely that a biomarker discovery approach targeting the cancer stem cell compartment may in the future yield diagnostic and prognostic panels with the highest accuracy. Also, most reported studies have emphasized the potential diagnostic and prognostic value of autoantibodies against antigens in cancer epithelial cells, whereas autoantibodies identifying stromal tumor autoantigens, which are also potentially valuable diagnostic and prognostic markers, have not received a great deal of attention.

An ever increasing number of autoantibodies are being reported in numerous diseases of seemingly different etiology, including type 1 diabetes and many other diseases in which the common denominator seems to be autoimmunity.[146–149] There are important lines of evidence suggesting that autoantibodies in cancer sera are not epiphenomena and that they can significantly contribute to the early diagnosis and prognosis of cancer. Moreover, the study of tumor-associated humoral autoimmunity may offer novel insights into the early events driving cancer.

SUMMARY

Autoantibodies are extremely promising diagnostic and prognostic biomarkers of cancer, and have the potential to promote early diagnosis and to make a large impact by improving patient outcome and decreasing mortality. Moreover, autoantibodies may be useful reagents in the identification of subjects at risk for cancer, bearing premalignant tissue changes.

Great efforts are being made in many laboratories to validate diagnostic panels of autoantibodies with high sensitivity and specificity that could be useful in a clinical setting. It is likely that prospective studies of sufficiently large cohorts of patients and controls using high-throughput technology may allow the identification of biomarkers with diagnostic significance, and perhaps of discrete antigen phenotypes with clinical significance.

The identification of TAAs may also be essential for the development of anticancer vaccines, because autoantibodies found in cancer sera target molecules involved in signal transduction, cell-cycle regulation, cell proliferation, and apoptosis, playing important roles in carcinogenesis. On this basis, molecular studies of antigen-antibody systems in cancer promise to yield valuable information on the carcinogenic process. TAAs identified by serum antibodies in cancer sera can be natural immunogenic molecules, useful as targets for cancer immunotherapy.

An important problem encountered in the practice of medicine is the identification of healthy individuals in the general population who unknowingly are at high risk of developing cancer. For the rheumatologist, a related problem is the identification of those patients with rheumatic diseases who are at high risk for developing a malignant process. These problems encountered in the fields of cancer and the rheumatic diseases can in the future be helped by new diagnostic instruments based on antibodies. The need for promoting the early diagnosis of cancer is a recognized major public health problem in need of significant research support for the validation of multiple promising but inconclusive studies, with the intention of producing diagnostic panels of autoantibodies in various types of cancers. Cancer developing in patients with rheumatic diseases is also an important problem requiring prospective long-term follow-up studies of patients with rheumatic diseases, particularly because some of the new biologic therapies seem to increase the cancer risk. It is possible that a panel of autoantibodies common to patients with cancer and the rheumatic diseases may prove to be of value in the identification of those patients with ADs at high risk for neoplasms.

REFERENCES

1. Burnham TK. Antinuclear antibodies in patients with malignancies. Lancet 1972; 26:436.
2. Zuber M. Positive antinuclear antibodies in malignancies. Ann Rheum Dis 1992; 51:573–4.
3. Fernández Madrid F, Karvonen RL, Kraut MJ, et al. Autoimmunity to collagen in human lung cancer. Cancer Res 1996;56:21–126.
4. Fernández-Madrid F, VandeVord PJ, Yang X, et al. Antinuclear antibodies as potential markers of lung cancer. Clin Cancer Res 1999;5:1393–400.
5. Tomkiel JE, Alansari H, Tang N, et al. Autoimmunity to the Mr 32,000 subunit of replication protein A in breast cancer. Clin Cancer Res 2002;8:752–8.
6. Fernández Madrid F, Tomkiel J. Antinuclear antibodies as potential markers of lung cancer. In: Shoenfeld Y, Gershwin ME, editors. Cancer and autoimmunity. Amsterdam: Elsevier; 2000. p. 151–8.
7. Tan EM. Autoantibodies as reporters identifying aberrant cellular mechanisms in tumorigenesis. J Clin Invest 2001;108:1411–5.
8. Tan EM, Shi FD, Keck WM. Relative paradigms between autoantibodies in lupus and autoantibodies in cancer. Clin Exp Immunol 2003;134:169–77.
9. Tan EM. Antinuclear antibodies: diagnostic markers for autoimmune diseases and probes for cell biology. Adv Immunol 1989;44:93–151.
10. Reichlin M. Systemic lupus erythematosus. In: Rose NR, Mackay IR, editors. The autoimmune diseases. 3rd edition. San Diego: Acad. Press; 1998. p. 283–98.
11. Alspaugh M, Maddison PJ. Resolution of the identity of certain antigen-antibody systems in systemic lupus erythematosus and Sjögren's syndrome: an interlaboratory collaboration. Arthritis Rheum 1979;22:796–8.
12. Von Mühlen CA, Tan EM. Autoantibodies in the diagnosis of systemic rheumatic diseases. Semin Arthritis Rheum 1995;24:323–58.
13. Harley JB. Autoantibodies in systemic lupus erythematosus. In: Koopman WJ, editor. 13th edition, Arthritis and allied diseases. a text of rheumatology, vol. 2 1997. p. 347–60.
14. Sahin U, Tureci O, Schmitt H, et al. Human neoplasms elicit multiple specific immune responses in the autologous host. Proc Natl Acad Sci U S A 1995;92: 11810–3.
15. Chen YT. Identification of human tumor antigens by serological expression cloning: an online review on SEREX. Cancer Immunol 2004. Available at: http://www.cancerimmunity.org/SEREX/. Accessed March, 2004.

16. Fernández-Madrid F, Tang N, Alansari H, et al. Autoantibodies to annexin XI-A and other autoantigens in the diagnosis of breast cancer. Cancer Res 2004; 64:5089–96.

17. Fernández Madrid F. Autoantibodies in breast cancer sera: candidate biomarkers and reporters of tumorigenesis. Cancer Lett 2005;230:187–98.

18. Chatterjee M, Mohapatra S, Ionan A, et al. Diagnostic markers of ovarian cancer by high-throughput antigen cloning and detection on arrays. Cancer Res 2006; 66:1181–90.

19. Wang X, Yu J, Sreekumar A, et al. Autoantibody signatures in prostate cancer. N Engl J Med 2005;353:1224–35.

20. Lin HS, Talwar HS, Tarca AL, et al. Autoantibody approach for serum-based detection of head and neck cancer. Cancer Epidemiol Biomarkers Prev 2007; 16:2396–405.

21. Zhong L, Coe SP, Stromberg AJ, et al. Profiling tumor-associated antibodies for early detection of non-small cell lung cancer. J Thorac Oncol 2006;1:513–9.

22. Hanash S. Disease proteomics. Nature 2003;422:226–32.

23. Hanash S. Harnessing the immune response for cancer detection. Cancer Epidemiol Biomarkers Prev 2011;20:569–70.

24. Zhang JY, Casiano CA, Peng XX, et al. Enhancement of antibody detection in cancer using panel of recombinant tumor-associated antigens. Cancer Epidemiol Biomarkers Prev 2003;12:136–43.

25. Storr SJ, Chakrabarti J, Barnes A, et al. Use of autoantibodies in breast cancer screening and diagnosis. Expert Rev Anticancer Ther 2006;6:1215–23.

26. Boyle P, Chapman CJ, Holdenrieder S, et al. Clinical validation of an autoantibody test for lung cancer. Ann Oncol 2011;22:383–9.

27. Shoenfeld Y, Ben-Yehuda O, Napartstek Y, et al. The detection of a common idiotype of anti-DNA antibodies in the sera of patients with monoclonal gammopathies. J Clin Immunol 1986;6:194–204.

28. Shoenfeld Y, El-Roeiy A, Ben-Yehuda O, et al. Detection of anti-histone activity in sera of patients with monoclonal gammopathies. Clin Immunol Immunopathol 1987;42:250–8.

29. Abou-Shakrah M, Krupp M, Argov S, et al. The detection of anti-Sm-RNP activity in sera of patients with monoclonal gammopathies. Clin Exp Immunol 1989;75: 349–53.

30. Syrigos KN, Charalambopoulos A, Pliarchopoulou K, et al. The prognostic significance of autoantibodies against dsDNA in patients with colorectal adenocarcinoma. Anticancer Res 2000;20:4351–3.

31. Lleo A, Invernizzi P, Gao B, et al. Definition of human autoimmunity-autoantibodies versus autoimmune disease. Autoimmun Rev 2010;9:A259–66.

32. Rugienė R, Dadonienė J, Aleknavičius E, et al. Prevalence of paraneoplastic rheumatic syndromes and their antibody profile among patients with solid tumours. Clin Rheumatol 2011;30:373–80.

33. Racanelli V, Prete M, Minoia C, et al. Rheumatic disorders as paraneoplastic syndromes. Autoimmun Rev 2008;7:352–8.

34. McCarty GA. Autoimmunity and malignancy. Med Clin North Am 1985;69: 599–615.

35. Abu-Shakra M, Buskila D, Ehrenfeld M, et al. Cancer and autoimmunity: autoimmune and rheumatic features in patients with malignancies. Ann Rheum Dis 2001;60:433–41.

36. Carsons S. The association of malignancy with rheumatic and connective tissue diseases. Semin Oncol 1997;24:360–72.

37. Ehrenfeld M, Shoenfeld Y. Malignancies and autoimmune rheumatic diseases. J Clin Rheumatol 2001;7:47–50.

38. Szekanecz Z, Szekanecz E, Bakó G, et al. Malignancies in autoimmune rheumatic diseases—a mini-review. Gerontology 2011;57:3–10.

39. Dinarello CA, Mier JW. Lymphokines. N Engl J Med 1987;317:940–5.

40. Nicolini A, Carpi A, Rossi G. Cytokines in breast cancer. Cytokine Growth Factor Rev 2006;17:325–37.

41. Smyth MJ, Cretney E, Kershaw MH, et al. Cytokines in cancer immunity and immunotherapy. Immunol Rev 2004;202:275–93.

42. Nzula S, Going JJ, Scott DI. Antigen-driven clonal proliferation, somatic hypermutation, and selection of B lymphocytes infiltrating human ductal breast carcinomas. Cancer Res 2003;63:3275–80.

43. De Visser KE, Koretz LV, Coussens LM. De novo carcinogenesis promoted by chronic inflammation is B lymphocyte dependent. Cancer Cell 2008;7:411–23.

44. Hansen MH, Nielsen HV, Ditzel HJ. Translocation of an intracellular antigen to the antibody response elicited by tumor-infiltrating B cells. J Immunol 2002; 169:2701–11.

45. Coronella-Wood JA, Hersh EM. Naturally occurring B-cell responses to breast cancer. Cancer Immunol Immunother 2003;52:715–38.

46. Johansson M, Denardo DG, Coussens LM. Polarized immune responses differentially regulate cancer development. Immunol Rev 2008;222:145–54.

47. DeNardo DG, Coussens LM. Inflammation and breast cancer. Balancing immune response: crosstalk between adaptive and innate immune cells during breast cancer progression. Breast Cancer Res 2007;9:212.

48. Chapman CJ, Murray A, McElveen JE, et al. Autoantibodies in lung cancer: possibilities for early detection and subsequent cure. Thorax 2008;63:228–33.

49. Koziol JA, Zhang JY, Casiano CA, et al. Recursive partitioning as an approach to selection of immune markers for tumor diagnosis. Clin Cancer Res 2003;9: 5120–6.

50. Brichory F, Beer D, LeNaour F, et al. Proteomics-based identification of protein gene product 9.5 as a tumor antigen that induces a humoral immune response in lung cancer. Cancer Res 2001;61:7908–12.

51. Carlsson P, Olofsson SO, Bondjers G, et al. Molecular cloning of human apolipoprotein B cDNA. Nucleic Acids Res 1985;13:8813–26.

52. Ekins RP. Multi-analyte immunoassay. J Pharm Biomed Anal 1989;7:155–68.

53. Robinson WH, DiGennaro C, Hueber W, et al. Autoantigen microarrays for multiplex characterization of autoantibody responses. Nat Med 2002;8:295–301.

54. Lee KH. Proteomics: a technology-driven and technology-limited discovery science. Trends Biotechnol 2001;19:217–22.

55. Ge H. UPA, a universal protein array system for quantitative detection of protein-protein, protein-DNA, protein-RNA and protein-ligand interactions. Nucleic Acids Res 2000;28:e3.

56. Walter G, Büssow K, Cahill D, et al. Protein arrays for gene expression and molecular interaction screening. Curr Opin Microbiol 2000;3:298–302.

57. Ekins RP. Ligand assays: from electrophoresis to miniaturized microarrays. Clin Chem 1998;44:2015–30.

58. Lagarkova MA, Koroleva EP, Kuprash DV, et al. Evaluation of humoral response to tumor antigens using recombinant expression-based serological mini-arrays. Immunol Lett 2003;85:71–4.

59. Fernández Madrid F, Tang N, Alansari H, et al. Improved approach to identify cancer-associated autoantigens. Autoimmun Rev 2005;4:230–5.

60. Fernández Madrid F, Chen W, Tang N, et al. Autoantibodies in breast cancer identify proteins involved in self-renewal and epigenetic chromatin remodeling. Open Biomarkers J 2010;3:13–20.
61. D'Orsi CJ, Newell MS. On the frontline of screening for breast cancer. Semin Oncol 2011;38:119–27.
62. National Lung Screening Trial Research Team, Aberle DR, Adams AM, et al. Reduced lung-cancer mortality with low-dose computed tomographic screening. N Engl J Med 2011;365:395–409.
63. Bei R, Masuelli L, Palumbo C, et al. A common repertoire of autoantibodies is shared by cancer and autoimmune disease patients: inflammation in their induction and impact on tumor growth. Cancer Lett 2009;281:8–23.
64. Saif MW, Zalonis A, Syrigos K. The clinical significance of autoantibodies in gastrointestinal malignancies: an overview. Expert Opin Biol Ther 2007;7:493–507.
65. Whitehouse JM, Holborow EJ. Smooth muscle antibody in malignant disease. Br Med J 1971;4:511–3.
66. Wasserman J, Glas U, Blomgren H. Autoantibodies in patients with carcinoma of the breast. Clin Exp Immunol 1975;19:417–22.
67. Imai H, Nakano Y, Ochs RH, et al. Nuclear antigens and autoantibodies in hepatocellular carcinoma and other malignancies. Am J Pathol 1992;140:859–70.
68. Solans-Laqué R, Pérez-Bocanegra C, Salud-Salvia A, et al. Clinical significance of antinuclear antibodies in malignant diseases: association with rheumatic and connective tissue paraneoplastic syndromes. Lupus 2004;13:159–64.
69. Friou GJ. Clinical application of a test for lupus globulin-nucleohistone interaction using fluorescent antibody. Yale J Biol Med 1958;31:40–7.
70. Rondeel JM. Immunofluorescence versus ELISA for the detection of antinuclear antigens. Expert Rev Mol Diagn 2002;2:226–32.
71. Jitsukawa T, Nakajima S, Junka U, et al. Detection of anti-nuclear antibodies from patients with systemic rheumatic diseases by ELISA using HEp-2 cell nuclei. J Clin Lab Anal 1991;5:49–53.
72. Keren DF. Antinuclear antibody testing. Clin Lab Med 2002;22:447–74.
73. Martins TB, Burlingame R, von Muhlen CA, et al. Evaluation of multiplexed fluorescent microsphere immunoassay for detection of autoantibodies to nuclear antigens. Clin Diagn Lab Immunol 2004;11:1054–9.
74. Li QZ, Karp DR, Quan J, et al. Risk factors for ANA positivity in healthy persons. Arthritis Res Ther 2011;13:R38.
75. Pisetsky DS. Antinuclear antibodies in healthy people: the tip of autoimmunity's iceberg? Arthritis Res Ther 2011;13:109.
76. Ackerman LS. Sex hormones and the genesis of autoimmunity. Arch Dermatol 2006;142:371–6.
77. Cutolo M. Estrogen metabolites: increasing evidence for their role in rheumatoid arthritis and systemic lupus erythematosus. J Rheumatol 2004;31:419–21.
78. Treurniet RA, Bergitjk EC, Baelde JJ, et al. Gender-related influences on the development of chronic graft-versus-host disease induced experimental lupus nephritis. Clin Exp Immunol 1993;91:442–8.
79. Marriott I, Huet-Hudson YM. Sexual dimorphism in innate immune responses to infectious organisms. Immunol Res 2006;34:177–92.
80. Libert C, Dejager I, Pinheiro I. The X chromosome in immune functions: when a chromosome makes a difference. Nat Rev Immunol 2010;10:594–604.
81. Arbuckle MR, McClain MT, Rubertone MV, et al. Development of autoantibodies before the clinical onset of systemic lupus erythematosus. N Engl J Med 2003; 349:1526–33.

82. Frenkel K, Karkoszka J, Kato J, et al. Systemic biomarkers of cancer risk. Cancer Detect Prev 1996;20:234.

83. Frenkel K, Karkoszka J, Glassman T, et al. Serum autoantibodies recognizing 5-hydroxymethyl-2′-deoxyuridine, an oxidized DNA base, as biomarkers of cancer risk in women. Cancer Epidemiol Biomarkers Prev 1998;7:49–57.

84. Shiel WC, Jason M. The diagnostic associations of patients with antinuclear antibodies referred to a community rheumatologist. J Rheumatol 1989;16:782–5.

85. Gómez-Puerta JA, Cervera R, Espinosa G, et al. Antiphospholipid antibodies associated with malignancies: clinical and pathological characteristics of 120 patients. Semin Arthritis Rheum 2006;35:322–32.

86. Cervera R, Piette JC, Font J, et al. Antiphospholipid syndrome: Clinical and immunological manifestations and patterns of disease expression in a cohort of 1,000 patients. Arthritis Rheum 2002;46:1019–27.

87. Zuckerman E, Toubi E, Dov Golan T, et al. Increased thromboembolic incidence in anti-cardiolipin-positive patients with malignancy. Br J Cancer 1995;72:447–51.

88. De Meis E, Monteiro RQ, Levy RA. Lung adenocarcinoma and antiphospholipid antibodies. Autoimmun Rev 2009;8:529–32.

89. Armas JB, Dantas J, Mendonça D, et al. Anticardiolipin and antinuclear antibodies in cancer patients—a case control study. Clin Exp Rheumatol 2000;18:227–32.

90. Miesbach W, Scharrer I, Asherson RA. High titres of IgM-antiphospholipid antibodies are unrelated to pathogenicity in patients with non-Hodgkin's lymphoma. Clin Rheumatol 2007;26:95–7.

91. Lossos I, Bogomolski-Yahalom V, Matzner Y. Anticardiolipin antibodies in acute myeloid leukemia: prevalence and clinical significance. Am J Hematol 1998;57:139–43.

92. Font C, Vidal L, Espinosa G, et al. Solid cancer, antiphospholipid antibodies, and venous thromboembolism. Autoimmun Rev 2011;10:222–7.

93. Sène D, Piette JC, Cacoub P. Antiphospholipid antibodies, antiphospholipid syndrome and infections. Autoimmun Rev 2008;7:272–7.

94. Ostrowski RA, Robinson JA. Antiphospholipid antibody syndrome and autoimmune diseases. Hematol Oncol Clin North Am 2008;22:53–65.

95. Crawford LV, Pim DC, Bulbrook RD. Detection of antibodies against the cellular protein p53 in sera from patients with breast cancer. Int J Cancer 1982;30:403–8.

96. Caron de Fromentel C, May-Levin F, Mouriesse H, et al. Presence of circulating antibodies against cellular protein p53 in a notable proportion of children with B-cell lymphoma. Int J Cancer 1987;39:185–9.

97. Soussi T. p53 Antibodies in the sera of patients with various types of cancer: a review. Cancer Res 2000;60:1777–88.

98. Sionov RV, Haupt Y. Apoptosis by p53: mechanisms, regulation, and clinical implication. Springer Semin Immunopathol 1998;19:345–62.

99. Lane DP. p53, guardian of the genome. Nature 1992;358:15–6.

100. Winter SF, Minna JD, Johnson BE, et al. Development of antibodies against p53 in lung cancer patients appears to be dependent on the type of p53 mutation. Cancer Res 1992;52:4168–74.

101. Cesare E, Previti M, Lombardo F, et al. Serum anti-p53 autoantibodies in patients with type 1 diabetes. Ann Clin Lab Sci 2001;31:253–8.

102. Kovacs B, Patel A, Hershey JN, et al. Antibodies against p53 in sera from patients with systemic lupus erythematosus and other rheumatic diseases. Arthritis Rheum 1997;40:980–5.

103. Fenton CL, Patel A, Tuttle RM, et al. Autoantibodies to p53 in sera of patients with autoimmune thyroid disease. Ann Clin Lab Sci 2000;30:179–83.
104. Chauhan R, Handa R, Das TP, et al. Over-expression of TATA binding protein (TBP) and p53 and autoantibodies to these antigens are features of systemic sclerosis, systemic lupus erythematosus and overlap syndromes. Clin Exp Immunol 2004;136:574–84.
105. Maehara Y, Kakeji Y, Watanabe A, et al. Clinical implications of serum anti-p53 antibodies for patients with gastric carcinoma. Cancer 1999;85:302–8.
106. Kressner U, Glimelius B, Bergstrom R, et al. Increased serum p53 antibody levels indicate poor prognosis in patients with colorectal cancer. Br J Cancer 1998;77:1848–51.
107. Werner JA, Gottschlich S, Folz BJ, et al. p53 serum antibodies as prognostic indicator in head and neck cancer. Cancer Immunol Immunother 1997;44:112–6.
108. Lenner P, Wiklund F, Emdin SO, et al. Serum antibodies against p53 in relation to cancer risk and prognosis in breast cancer: a population-based epidemiological study. Br J Cancer 1999;79:927–32.
109. Lubin R, Zalcman G, Bouchet L, et al. Serum p53 antibodies as early markers of lung cancer. Nat Med 1995;1:701–2.
110. Yamauchi T, Naoe T, Kurosawa Y, et al. Autoantibodies to c-myc nuclear protein products in autoimmune disease. Immunology 1990;69:117–20.
111. Doyle GA, Bordeaux-Heller JM, Coulthard S, et al. Amplification in human breast cancer of a gene encoding a c-myc mRNA binding protein. Cancer Res 2000; 60:2756–9.
112. Ben-Mahrez K, Sorokine I, Thierry D, et al. Circulating antibodies against c-myc oncogene product in sera of colorectal cancer patients. Int J Cancer 1990;46:35–8.
113. Donner P, Greiser-Wilke I, Moelling K. Nuclear localization and DNA binding of the transforming gene product of avian myelocytomatosis virus. Nature 1982; 296:262–9.
114. Mimori T, Ohosone Y, Hama N, et al. Isolation and characterization of the 80-kDa subunit protein of the human autoantigen Ku (p70/p80) recognized by antibodies from patients with scleroderma-polymyositis overlap syndrome. Proc Natl Acad Sci U S A 1990;87:1777–81.
115. Sigurgeirsson B, Lindelöf B, Edhag O, et al. Risk of cancer in patients with dermatomyositis or polymyositis. N Engl J Med 1992;326:363–7.
116. Targoff IN. Humoral immunity in polymyositis/dermatomyositis. J Invest Dermatol 1993;100:116S–23S.
117. Love LA, Leff RL, Fraser DD, et al. A new approach to the classification of idiopathic inflammatory myopathy: myositis specific autoantibodies define useful homogeneous patient groups. Medicine 1991;70:360–74.
118. Belizna C, Henrion D, Beucher A, et al. Anti-Ku antibodies: clinical, genetic and diagnostic insights. Autoimmun Rev 2010;9:691–4.
119. Burgman P, Ouyang H, Peterson S, et al. Heat inactivation of Ku autoantigen: possible role in hyperthermic radiosensitization. Cancer Res 1997;57:2847–50.
120. Lieber MR, Ma Y, Pannicke U, et al. The mechanism of vertebrate nonhomologous DNA end joining and its role in V(D)J recombination. DNA Repair (Amst) 2004;3:817–26.
121. Foidart JM, Abe S, Martin GR, et al. Antibodies to type II collagen in relapsing polychondritis. N Engl J Med 1978;299:1203–7.
122. Rowley MJ, Williamson DJ, Mackay IR. Evidence for local synthesis of antibodies to denatured collagen in the synovium in rheumatoid arthritis. Arthritis Rheum 1987;30:1420–5.

123. Tarkowski A, Klareskog L, Carlsten H, et al. Secretion of antibodies to types I and II collagen by synovial tissue cells in patients with rheumatoid arthritis. Arthritis Rheum 1989;32:1087–92.

124. Bhowmick N, Neilson E, Moses H. Stromal fibroblasts in cancer initiation and progression. Nature 2004;432:332–7.

125. De Wever O, Mareel M. Role of tissue stroma in cancer cell invasion. J Pathol 2003;200:429–47.

126. Tokumitsu H, Mizutani A, Minami H, et al. A calcyclin-associated protein is a newly identified member of the Ca^{2+}/phospholipid-binding proteins, annexin family. J Biol Chem 1992;267:8919–24.

127. Erdile L, Wold MS, Kelly TJ. The primary structure of the 32 kDa subunit of human replication protein A. J Biol Chem 1990;265:3177–82.

128. Seogerson L, Moldave K. Characterization of the interaction of aminoacyltransferase II with ribosomes. Binding of transferase II and translocation of peptidyl transfer ribonucleic acid. J Biol Chem 1968;243:5354–60.

129. Schneider JA, Raeburn S, Maxwell ES. Translocase activity in the aminoacyltransferase II fraction from rat liver. Biochem Biophys Res Commun 1968;33:177–81.

130. Jorgensen CS, Levantino G, Houen G, et al. Determination of autoantibodies to annexin XI in systemic autoimmune diseases. Lupus 2000;9:515–20.

131. Misaki Y, Pruijn GJ, van derKemp AW. The 56K autoantigen is identical to human annexin XI. J Biol Chem 1994;269:4240–6.

132. Garcia Lozano R, Gonzalez Escribano F, Sanchez Roman J, et al. Presence of antibodies to different subunit of replication protein A in autoimmune sera. Proc Natl Acad Sci U S A 1995;92:5116–20.

133. Alberdi F, Dadone J, Ryazanov A, et al. Cross-reaction of lupus anti-dsDNA antibodies with protein translation factor EF-2. Clin Immunol 2001;98:293–300.

134. Talal N. Benign and malignant lymphoid proliferation in autoimmunity. Recent Results Cancer Res 1978;64:288–91.

135. Anaya JM, McGuff HS, Banks PM, et al. Clinicopathological factors relating malignant lymphoma with Sjogren's syndrome. Semin Arthritis Rheum 1996;25:337–46.

136. Yeatman TJ, Updyke TV, Kaetzel MA, et al. Expression of annexins on the surfaces of non-metastatic and metastatic human and rodent cells. Clin Exp Metastasis 1993;11:37–44.

137. Chetcuti A, Margan SH, Russel P, et al. Loss of annexin II heavy and light chains in prostate cancer and its precursors. Cancer Res 2001;61:6331–4.

138. Brichori FM, Misek DE, Yim AM, et al. An immune response manifested by the common occurrence of annexins I and II autoantibodies and high circulating levels of IL-6 in lung cancer. Proc Natl Acad Sci U S A 2001;98:9824–9.

139. Parmer TG, Ward MD, Yurkow EJ, et al. Activity and regulation by growth factors of calmodulin-dependent protein kinase III (elongation factor 2-kinase) in human breast cancer. Br J Cancer 1999;79:59–64.

140. Coussens LM, Werb Z. Inflammation and cancer. Nature 2002;420:860–7.

141. Alberto Mantovani A, Allavena P, Sica A. Cancer-related inflammation. Nature 2008;454:436–44.

142. Franklin WA, Gazdar A, Haney J, et al. Widely dispersed p53 mutations in respiratory epithelium. J Clin Invest 1997;100:2133–7.

143. Lapidot T, Sirard C, Vormoor J, et al. A cell initiating human acute myeloid leukemia after transplantation into SCID mice. Nature 1994;367:645–8.

144. Sell S, Pierce GB. Maturation arrest of stem cell differentiation is a common pathway for the cellular origin of teratocarcinomas and epithelial cancers. Lab Invest 1994;70:6–22.

145. Wicha MS, Liu S, Dontu G. Cancer stem cells: an old idea-a paradigm shift. Cancer Res 2006;66:383–90.
146. Eisenbarth GS. Type I diabetes mellitus. N Engl J Med 1986;314:1360–8.
147. Fernando MM, Stevens CR, Walsh EC, et al. Defining the role of the MHC in autoimmunity: a review and pooled analysis. PLoS Genet 2008;4:e1000024.
148. Sawcer S, Compston A. Multiple sclerosis: light at the end of the tunnel. Eur J Hum Genet 2006;14:257–8.
149. Todd JA. Genetic control of autoimmunity in type 1 diabetes. Immunol Today 1990;11:122–9.

Rheumatic Manifestations of Primary and Metastatic Bone Tumors and Paraneoplastic Bone Disease

Christian A. Waimann, MD*, Huifang Lu, MD, PhD,
Maria E. Suarez Almazor, MD, PhD

KEYWORDS

- Bone tumors • Paraneoplastic syndromes
- Rheumatic manifestations • Osteoporosis • Osteomalacia
- Osteonecrosis

Musculoskeletal symptoms are usually the first manifestation of bone tumors. These symptoms can simulate a wide range of rheumatic disorders, delaying tumor diagnosis and therefore the probability of cure.[1,2] Tumors can affect the bone through both direct and indirect mechanisms. Primary bone tumors and metastases (**Box 1**) are responsible for direct effects, whereas paraneoplastic syndromes, metabolic changes, and therapeutic toxicity result in indirect effects on the bone. In this article, the authors first review the clinical presentation of primary and metastatic bone tumors, with particular emphasis on differential diagnosis with other musculoskeletal conditions and atypical symptoms that should alert clinicians of an underlying malignancy. They then summarize the most common paraneoplastic syndromes affecting bone. The metabolic changes of bone caused by cancer and cancer treatment are also described.

Disclosures: C.A.W has nothing to disclose; M.S.A. received honorarium from Zimmer; H.L. received research funding from Genentech.

Section of Rheumatology, Department of General Internal Medicine, The University of Texas at MD Anderson Cancer Center, 1515 Holcombe Boulevard, Unit 1465, Houston, TX 77030, USA
* Corresponding author.
E-mail address: christianwaimann@gmail.com

Box 1
Bone tumors, miscellaneous and tumorlike bone lesions

Primary bone malignancies

    Osteosarcoma

    Ewing sarcoma

    Chondrosarcoma

    Other histologies: Fibrosarcoma; malignant fibrous histiocytoma, hemangiosarcoma, malignant hemangioendothelioma, malignant epithelioid hemangioendothelioma, malignant chondroblastoma, malignant in giant cell tumor of bone, adamantinoma of long bone, malignant odontogenic tumor, malignant ameloblastoma, chordoma, leiomyosarcoma, liposarcoma

Hematopoietic tumors

    Plasma cell myeloma

    Lymphoma

Metastatic malignancy

Benign bone tumors

    Bone-forming tumors: osteoma, osteoid osteoma, osteoblastoma

    Giant cell tumor

    Vascular tumors: hemangioma, lymphangioma, glomus tumor

    Other connective tissue tumors: desmoplastic fibroma, fibrous histiocytoma, lipoma, leiomyoma, neurilemoma, neurofibroma

    Cartilage-forming tumors: chondroma, enchondroma, osteochondroma, chondroblastoma, chondromyxoid fibroma

Miscellaneous lesions

    Solitary bone cyst

    Aneurysmal bone cyst

    Fibrous dysplasia

    Osteofibrous dysplasia or ossifying fibroma

    Metaphyseal fibrous defect or nonossifying fibroma

    Langerhans cell histiocytosis

Tumorlike lesions

    Brown tumor of hyperparathyroidism

    Reparative granuloma

    Chronic osteomyelitis (Brodie abscess)

    Acute osteomyelitis

    Bone infarct

Data from Dorfman H, Czerniak B, Kotz R, et al. WHO classification of bone tumours. In: Fletcher C, Krishnan Unni K, Mertens F, editors. Pathology and genetics of tumours of soft tissue and bone. Lyon (France): IARCPress; 2006. p. 227–32.

BONE TUMORS
Epidemiology

Primary bone and joint cancers represent only 0.2% of all cancers in people older than 20 years but are responsible for more than 5% of all malignancies in the younger population.[3–5] The peak incidence is between ages 10 and 20 years when these cancers account for 8% of all cancers, as the fourth cause of malignancy, only behind lymphoma, leukemia, and nervous system–related tumors.[5] Osteosarcoma, Ewing sarcoma, and chondrosarcoma are responsible for approximately 80% of all primary bone and joint cancers, the first 2 being the most prevalent cancers in children, whereas chondrosarcoma is the most common in older populations (**Fig. 1**).[3,6] After age 40 years, most bone tumors are metastatic, most commonly from breast, prostate, thyroid, lung, and renal carcinomas. Postmortem examination of patients dying from these cancers revealed bone metastases in 73%, 68%, 42%, 36%, and 35% of the cases, respectively.[7]

Multiple myeloma is the most frequent hematopoietic neoplasm of the bone and should be included in the differential diagnosis of every patient older than 40 years with multiple osteolytic bone lesions.[4] Primary bone lymphomas are uncommon and represent only 2% of all lymphomas. However, 20% of patients with lymphoma will develop secondary invasion of the bone during the course of their disease.[8,9]

Unlike bone cancer, the true incidence of benign bone tumors and tumorlike lesions is unknown, with a prevalence of about one-half of that of all bone tumors combined. These conditions usually develop during childhood but can remain asymptomatic or manifest themselves later in life.[10] The most frequent benign bone tumors include osteoid osteoma, osteochondromas, enchondromas, and hemangiomas of the spine (**Table 1**).[11] Giant cell tumor is another relatively common bone neoplasm, accounting for 8% of primary bone tumors in Western populations[12] but almost 20% in Asians.[13] The peak incidence of this tumor is between 15 and 30 years of age, but this tumor can also occur later in life.[12] Giant cell tumor is considered semimalignant, with a clinical

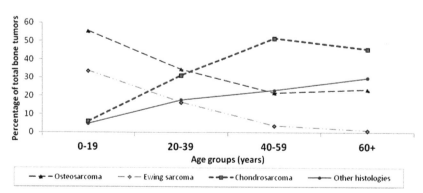

Fig. 1. Relative frequencies of bone sarcomas by histology type and age group. (*Data from* Lewis DR, Ries LAG. Cancers of the Bone and Joint. In: Ries LAG, Young JL, Keel GE, et al, editors. SEER Survival Monograph: Cancer Survival Among Adults: U.S. SEER Program, 1988–2001, Patient and Tumor Characteristics. Bethesda (MD): National Cancer Institute, SEER Program, NIH Pub. No. 07-6215; 2007. p. 81–8; and Gurney JG, Swensen AR, Bulterys M. Malignant Bone Tumors. In: Ries LAG, Smith MA, Gurney JG, et al, editors. Cancer Incidence and Survival among Children and Adolescents: United States SEER Program 1975–1995. Bethesda (MD): National Cancer Institute, SEER Program. NIH Pub. No. 99-4649; 1999. p. 99–110.)

Table 1
Clinical features of most commons benign bone tumors and tumorlike lesions

	Frequency	Typical Clinical Presentation
Benign tumors		
Cartilaginous lesions		
Osteochondroma	33% of benign bone tumors[a]	Usually located in long bones but may also affect posterior elements of the spine. Only develop symptoms when the tumor compresses nearby structures. Surgical excision is indicated when symptoms are present. Recurrence rate is low
Enchondroma	16% of benign bone tumors[a]	Long bones lesions are usually asymptomatic. Patients with involvement of small bones of hands and feet frequently present fractures and pain. Curettage is indicated only if symptoms are present. Recurrence is extremely rare
Bone-forming lesions		
Osteoid osteoma	13% of benign bone tumors[a]	The most frequent sites are femur and tibia but any bone can be affected. Patients classically manifest with intense bone pain that typically worsens at night and presents a fast and excellent response to nonsteroidal antiinflammatory drugs. Treatment includes complete removal of the nidus. Recurrence can be seen only in cases of incomplete removal
Vascular tumors		
Hemangioma	10%–12% of general population[b]	Generally located on spine or skull. Asymptomatic. On rare occasions, patients can develop neurologic symptoms due to spinal cord compression
Giant cell tumor	22% of benign bone tumors,[a] 7.8% of primary bone tumors	Usually located in long bones, especially distal femur and proximal tibia. Patients often present pain and swelling. Clinical manifestation depends on tumor aggressiveness and location. Surgery is mandatory. Recurrence rate varies from 25%–50%

Tumorlike lesions		
Cyst lesion		
Aneurysmal bone cyst	12% of benign bone tumors[a]	Rapidly blood-filled cyst. Located on long bones and posterior elements of the spine. Patients experience pain associated with rapidly enlarging mass. Compression symptoms can be seen, especially when the spine is involved. Curettage is indicated. Recurrence is rare
Simple bone cyst	Unknown	Fluid-filled cyst. Located in femur and humerus in children and calcaneus and ilium in adults. Asymptomatic. Treatment is indicated only when symptoms are present and includes fluid aspiration and steroids injection
Fibrous lesions		
Metaphyseal fibrous defect	35% of children between ages 4–8 y	Metaphysis of long bones. Usually asymptomatic and rarely produce pain. A pathologic fracture may be the first and sole manifestation. Treatment is only required in cases with high risk of fracture and includes curettage with bone grafting
Fibrous dysplasia	Unknown	Bone replacement by fibrous tissue. Mono-ostotic or polyostotic (McCune-Albright syndrome). The most common site is the femoral neck. Generally asymptomatic. Pathologic fracture may be the first and sole manifestation. Treatment included curettage and stabilization if necessary. Recurrence is frequent. Bisphosphonates could be an option

[a] Surgical series from Mayo clinic files. True incidence is unknown because patients are often asymptomatic and biopsy and surgery are not performed.
[b] Based on autopsy results.
Data from Unni KK, Inwards CY, Bridge JA, et al. Tumor of the bones and joints. AFIP Atlas of tumor pathology. vol. 2. Washington, DC: ARP press; 2005; and Robbins LR, Fountain EM. Hemangioma of cervical vertebras with spinal-cord compression. N Engl J Med 1958;258(14):685–87.

presentation varying from a well-defined intraosseous lesion to an aggressive lesion that breaks the cortex and extends to soft tissues.[14] This tumor has the potential to metastasize, mostly to the lung.[15]

Tumorlike bone lesions are nonneoplastic conditions that can occur as solitary or multiple bone lesions. The most frequent lesions in this group include metaphyseal fibrous defects and fibrous dysplasia. These fibrous lesions are characterized by fibrous replacement of bone and can result in pain, deformity, and spontaneous fractures.[11,16] Other common tumorlike lesions are cysts, which include unicameral or simple bone cysts and aneurysmal bone cysts (see **Table 1**).

Clinical Manifestations of Bone Tumors

Benign bone tumors are usually asymptomatic findings on a simple radiograph performed for other reasons. However, depending on the tumor location, extension, aggressiveness, and patient age, these tumors can cause joint effusion, limited mobility, spontaneous fractures, neurovascular compressions, deformities, or growth defects (eg, extremity disparities, scoliosis) (see **Table 1**).[16,17] Bone pain, an enlarging mass, and constitutional symptoms are considered the 3 cardinal signs and symptoms of malignant bone tumors. In addition, mass effects and system-specific symptoms can occur depending on the location of the tumor.

Pain
Pain is generally the first manifestation of bone tumors.[18] Initially, it is mild and intermittent, with higher intensity at night and during exercise. As the disease progresses, the pain becomes more severe, often requiring higher doses of analgesics. Osteoid osteoma is a benign bone-forming tumor. The tumor is rich in prostaglandins, and patients usually develop intense bone pain with a characteristically fast and excellent response to nonsteroidal antiinflammatory drugs (NSAIDs), usually within 20 to 25 minutes. This rapid response to NSAIDs plus the finding of the classical nidus (small radiolucent mass with well-defined surrounding sclerosis) on conventional radiography is usually sufficient for the diagnosis.[19]

Enlarging mass
An enlarging mass is usually a late manifestation of bone tumors, only evident when the tumor enlarges the bone or extends to extraosseous tissues. Clinical features favoring suspicion of an underlying malignancy are rapid growth, hyperthermia, skin ulceration, and adhesion to surrounding tissues. On the other hand, benign lesions are generally localized and do not adhere to skin or surrounding tissue.[17]

Joint effusion
Tumors adjacent to the joint, including epiphyseal and metaphyseal neoplasms, may cause joint effusion. The presence of an effusion with concomitant joint stiffness can be misleading, suggesting a diagnosis of inflammatory rheumatic disease, especially in pediatric populations.[20]

Limited mobility
Different factors can cause a decrease in joint mobility in patients with bone tumors, including pain, muscle atrophy or spasm, joint effusion, and large tumoral mass.

Pathologic fractures
Pathologic fractures are usually a late manifestation of malignant bone tumors.[21] In contrast, benign lesions are generally asymptomatic, but sometimes a pathologic fracture might be their initial and sole manifestation.[16]

Constitutional symptoms

Ewing sarcoma is the most common primary bone tumor associated with constitutional symptoms. Weight loss, fever, or anemia is present in 20% of the cases.[22] These manifestations often are similar to those seen in subacute osteomyelitis, which needs to be considered as a differential diagnosis. Both conditions can present with fever, anemia, weight loss, an elevated erythrosedimentation rate, bone and soft tissue mass, and increased radionuclide uptake on nuclear scan. However, unlike in osteomyelitis, culture results are negative in Ewing sarcoma.

Neurologic symptoms

Both malignant (eg, Ewing sarcoma, metastases) and benign lesions (eg, osteoid osteoma, osteoblastoma) can involve the spine, including the sacrum. Patients may develop a wide range of neurologic manifestations, including lumbago; sciatica; pain in the hips and buttocks; radiculopathy; and, in more severe cases, spinal cord compression.[1,23,24] The skull can also be affected by bone tumors (eg, multiple myeloma, enchondromatosis multiple), resulting in headache and, depending on the location, cranial nerve palsy. Occasionally, tumors of the skull might be misdiagnosed as giant cell arteritis.[25] The eosinophilic granuloma of bone has an especial avidity for the skull. Depending on tumor location, patients with this condition may develop jaw pain, proptosis, otitis refractory to treatment, and central nervous system involvement (especially diabetes insipidus).[26]

Role of Imaging in the Diagnosis and Management of Bone Tumors

In all patients with unexplained bone symptoms, a plain radiograph of the affected area is mandatory.[27,28] This simple study allows to easily confirm the diagnosis of some benign tumors (eg, metaphysical fibrous defect, fibrous dysplasia, and simple bone cysts) without further studies.[10] However, in a large proportion of patients, more advanced imaging techniques are needed, including computed tomography (CT), magnetic resonance imaging (MRI), radionuclide bone scans, and/or positron emission tomography (PET).[29]

A proper radiologic evaluation of a bone lesion should include a description of the pattern of bone destruction, tumor margins, periosteal reaction, lesion opacity, mineralization, and trabecular pattern. These characteristics in addition to the patient's age and tumor location narrow the spectrum of possible diagnoses.[30]

Age

Peak age differs among various tumors.[16,30] In general, before age 5 years, a malignant tumor is often a metastatic neuroblastoma; between 5 and 30 years of age, it is frequently osteosarcoma or Ewing sarcoma; and, after 30 years, a metastasis or multiple myeloma.[17] Benign lesions develop mostly in young patients; however, they can remain asymptomatic for many years and become clinically evident at an older age.[16]

Tumor location

According to Miller,[30] tumor location can be stratified into 3 categories: skeletal (axial or appendicular), longitudinal (diaphyseal, metaphyseal, or epiphyseal), and transversal (medullary, juxtacortical, or cortical) (**Fig. 2**). In addition, some tumors are typically associated with particular locations, such as hemangiomas with vertebral bodies, aneurysmal bone cysts and osteoblastomas with the posterior elements of the spine, and simple bone cysts and intraosseous lipomas with the calcaneous.[30]

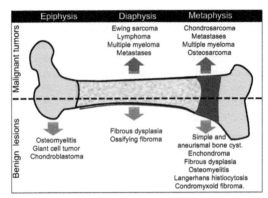

Fig. 2. Classification of tumors according to longitudinal location. (*Data from* Miller TT. Bone tumors and tumorlike conditions: analysis with conventional radiography. Radiology 2008;246(3):662–74.)

Patterns of bone destruction and lesion margins

Three classical destruction patterns have been described: geographic, moth eaten, and permeated (**Table 2**). Evidence suggestive of a nonaggressive lesion includes geographic pattern, narrow transition zone, well-defined borders, and sclerotic margins. On the other hand, a lesion has to be considered aggressive and potentially malignant when the images show a permeated or moth-eaten pattern, wide transition zone, ill-defined borders, and nonsclerotic margins.[31] These rules nevertheless can have exceptions because aggressive patterns can occasionally be seen in benign processes such as osteomyelitis or Langerhans cell histiocytosis.[17]

Periosteal reaction

The type of periosteal reaction depends on the rate of tumor progression. Nonaggressive lesions usually grow slowly and allow the periosteum to react, developing a thick, solid, and uniform callous. Instead, in aggressive tumors, the periosteum cannot adequately control the tumoral expansion and the radiographic images of the affected bone show perpendicular periosteal reaction (called hair-on-end or sunburst), cortical disruption, and Codman triangle, which is the disruption of an elevated periosteum "broken by the tumor," an image which can occasionally also be found in some benign lesions.[32]

Table 2	
Radiologic patterns of bone destruction	
Pattern	**Description**
Geographic	Focal lytic lesion
Type 1a	Well defined with sclerotic rim
Type 1b	Well defined, no sclerotic rim
Type 1c	Ill defined
Moth eaten (Type 2)	Patchy lytic holes
Permeated (Type 3)	Small lytic patchy lesions

Data from Miller TT. Bone tumors and tumorlike conditions: analysis with conventional radiography. Radiology 2008;246(3):662–74.

Lesion opacity

Lesion opacity is another radiologic feature often reported. Tumors can be predominantly sclerotic, predominantly lytic, or mixed.[33] This imaging feature is not always helpful in distinguishing between benign and malignant tumors because both can have lytic or sclerotic appearance. However, it can assist in identifying the origin of the primary tumor when metastatic disease is suspected (see "Multiple Lesions").

Mineralization pattern

Together with lesion opacity, the calcification pattern can suggest a diagnosis. Osteoid tumors often present a trabecular or cloud-like mineralization pattern. Calcification in a chondroid tumor has been described as ring-and-arcs, popcorn, and stippled or punctate.[34]

Multiple lesions

Multiple bone lesions seen in patients older than 40 years are highly suggestive of metastatic cancer.[33,35] These lesions are usually classified according to image opacity, with mixed patterns as the most common presentation (eg, breast cancer). Predominantly lytic metastases are seen in renal cell cancer, melanoma, and multiple myeloma, whereas predominantly sclerotic metastases are usually associated with prostate carcinoma, small cell lung cancer, and Hodgkin lymphoma.[7] Multiple lesions are not always malignant and can also be found in patients with multiple hemangiomas, hyperparathyroidism (Brown tumors), fibrous dysplasia, and multiple enchondromatosis. Osteopoikilosis is a rare hereditary disorder that also has to be considered in the presence of multiple sclerotic lesions. Characteristically, these patients develop multiple small radiodensities in bone metaphyses. In general, these patients remain asymptomatic throughout their lifetime.[36]

Advanced imaging techniques

MRI is considered the method of choice for the evaluation of bone and soft tissue masses. Its main advantages include better characterization of nonmineralized chondroid matrix, cysts, and lipomatous and vascular tissues, with high accuracy to define soft tissue involvement and extension and high sensitivity for detection of skip metastases distantly in the bone or transarticular in the opposite side of the adjacent joint.[11,29]

Although MRI is used more often than CT in the evaluation of bone tumors, the latter technique is sometimes useful to better characterize the involved bone, the mineralization pattern, and the definition of sclerotic margins.[37]

Radionuclide bone scans remain the standard imaging technique to evaluate the extent of metastatic bone disease. However, this technique has some disadvantages, including overestimation of tumor extension (high rate of false positives results) and a poor sensitivity to detect pure lytic lesions (eg, renal cell carcinoma metastases and multiple myeloma).[38–40]

New imaging techniques have been developed and evaluated during the past decade, such as whole-body MRI and PET. However, the precise role of these techniques in the diagnosis and evaluation of bone tumors and metastases needs to be established.[41,42]

Experienced radiologists can diagnose some benign bone tumors using 1 or more of these techniques with a degree of certainty, avoiding the need for biopsy.[17] However, when bone sarcoma is suspected because of radiologic features, rapid growth, or prolonged bone pain, prompt consultation with an orthopedic surgeon is mandatory for rapid diagnosis, biopsy, and therapeutic guidance.[27]

Prognosis and Treatment

The prognosis of patients with bone cancer has improved in the last decades.[5,6] Chondrosarcoma has the longest survival, followed by osteosarcoma and Ewing sarcoma (approximately 10, 7, and 5 years, respectively).[3,6]

In general, benign bone tumors have a good prognosis. However, depending on tumor aggressiveness and location, patients may develop complications that can occasionally be serious, including neurovascular compressions or growth defects in children. Local recurrence after treatment varies depending on tumor histology and type of treatment.

Malignant transformation of benign lesions is extremely rare except for osteochondromas and enchondromas. Osteochondromas are associated with an increased risk of bone cancer. In a retrospective study, 32 (5%) of 637 patients with bone tumors originating in the cartilage developed malignant transformation. Of the 32 patients, 14 had solitary osteochondroma, 10 had multiple osteochondromas, 6 had enchondromas, 1 had Ollier disease, and 1 had Maffucci syndrome.[43] Ollier disease is a rare condition, characterized by the presence of 2 or more enchondromas; when multiple soft tissue hemangiomas are also present, this syndrome is called Maffucci syndrome. These patients have an increased risk of developing chondrosarcoma.[25] Schwartz and colleagues[44] reported a series of 37 patients with Ollier disease and 7 with Maffucci disease. Ten patients developed chondrosarcoma, 1 osteosarcoma, and 5 cancer in other organs. Giant cell tumors can develop an aggressive course in approximately 20% of patients.[14] They are not considered to be malignant; however, in a retrospective review of 470 patients with giant cell tumors, 24 (5%) developed metastases, most often in the lung. Unlike metastatic sarcoma, giant cell metastases are less aggressive, and, in this series, no patients died during follow-up.[15]

PARANEOPLASTIC BONE SYNDROMES

There are 3 main paraneoplastic syndromes affecting the bone: humoral hypercalcemia of malignancy, hypertrophic osteoarthropathy (HOA), and tumor-induced osteomalacia.

Humoral Hypercalcemia of Malignancy

Humoral hypercalcemia of malignancy is a syndrome produced by ectopic secretion of parathyroid hormone–related protein (PTHrP). This hormone shares a similar N-terminal sequence with parathyroid hormone (PTH).[45] Burtis and colleagues[46] reported a series of 38 patients with hypercalcemia of malignancy. Nearly 80% of them showed high levels of PTHrP. In the remaining 8 patients, the hypercalcemia was attributed to osteolytic metastatic disease. Serum levels of PTHrP were low or undetectable in all 60 healthy controls. The most frequent etiology of humoral hypercalcemia was squamous cell cancer, accounting for 40% of the cases.

PTHrP binds to the PTH/PTHrP receptor resulting in similar metabolic effects as those of PTH, including increased bone reabsorption, reduced renal phosphorous reabsorption, and enhanced renal calcium retention. These metabolic changes result in the classical laboratory findings observed in primary hyperparathyroidism, including hypercalcemia, hypocalciuria, hypophosphatemia, and hyperphosphaturia. However, the effects of PTHrP and PTH are not entirely identical. Unlike what is seen in primary hyperparathyroidism, bone formation is totally suppressed in patients with humoral hypercalcemia of malignancy, and their levels of serum 1,25-dihydroxyvitamin D are usually low. The precise mechanisms accounting for these differences have not been clarified yet.[47,48]

Osteolytic metastases represent the second most common etiology of malignant hypercalcemia and account for 20% of the cases of malignant hypercalcemia, most frequently observed in patients with breast cancer or multiple myeloma. These patients can also have increased bone reabsorption caused by paracrine secretion of cytokines and PTHrP.[33,48,49] Other less frequent causes of hypercalcemia have to be considered in patients with cancer, including ectopic secretion of 1,25-dihydroxy-vitamin D or intact PTH by the tumoral cells.[50]

Hypercalcemia is usually a late complication of malignancies, carrying a high short-term mortality. Treatment depends on the severity of the hypercalcemia and the underlying tumor.[49]

HOA

HOA is a paraneoplastic syndrome characterized by digital clubbing and periostitis of tubular bones, with or without synovial effusion.[18] Digital clubbing results from the proliferation of the connective tissue between the nail matrix and the distal phalanx in the fingers and/or toes.[51] It can occur in isolation without periostitis in other bones. When advanced, clubbing can cause drumsticklike deformities that are typical and easy to recognize. At early stages, however, additional clinical tests might be needed for diagnosis, including[51]

1. Measurement of the nail fold angle as the nail exits the terminal phalanx. An angle greater than 180° is congruent with clubbing.[52]
2. Schamroth sign defined as "the absence of diamond shape window when the dorsal surfaces of opposite fingers are opposed."[53]
3. Measurement of the phalangeal depth ratio (distal phalange depth to interphalangeal finger depth). A ratio greater than 1 is considered positive. In addition, a digital index can be calculated summing the phalangeal depth ratios of the 10 fingers, and the diagnosis of clubbing is made when the result is greater than 10.

Periostitis is the hallmark of this syndrome. It generally affects distal long tubular bones, mostly the tibiae, fibulae, radii, ulnae, femora, and hummers. Periostitis can cause intense deep-seated bone pain, usually in the lower extremities, worsening with limb dependency and alleviated by leg elevation. Local tenderness may also be present. On conventional radiography, affected bones show symmetric unilamel-lated periosteal reaction, separated from the underlying bone by a radiolucent zone. Distal phalanges can exhibit bone proliferation and acro-osteolysis in more severe cases. In early stages, scintigraphy is more sensitive than conventional radiologic testing, with affected bones typically showing a pericortical radionuclide uptake line.[18,54]

A later manifestation of this syndrome is oligoarthritis or polyarthritis, often symmetric, painful, and affecting knees, ankles, elbows, wrists, and metacarpopha-langeal and proximal interphalangeal joints. The synovial fluid is characteristically noninflammatory.[54]

According to its etiology, HOA can be classified as primary or secondary (**Box 2**).[18,55] Primary HOA is a hereditary disorder caused by a mutation in the gene that encodes 15-hydroxyprostaglandin dehydrogenase.[56] This enzyme is essential for prostaglandin degradation. Because of the lack of this protein, these patients show high levels of prostaglandin E2 (PGE2) and develop the typical clinical features of HOA.[57] The precise link between PGE2 and HOA has not been elucidated, and the role of prostaglandins in secondary HOA is unclear. Among secondary causes, lung cancer has the highest risk of HOA. Sridhar and colleagues[58] reported a 29%

Box 2
Classification of HOA

Primary (or pachydermoperiostosis or Touraine-Solente-Golé syndrome)

Secondary

  Malignancy: non–small cell and oat cell lung carcinoma

  Pulmonary diseases: cystic fibrosis, chronic infection, pulmonary fibrosis, mesothelioma

  Cardiac diseases: right-to-left cardiac shunts

  Others: hepatic cirrhosis, inflammatory bowel diseases, esophageal carcinoma, POEMS syndrome (polyneuropathy, organomegaly, endocrinopathy, monoclonal protein, skin changes), rheumatologic diseases, vascular prosthesis infections, immune deficiency syndromes, and chronic infections.

Data from Nguyen S, Hojjati M. Review of current therapies for secondary hypertrophic pulmonary osteoarthropathy. Clin Rheumatol 2011;30(1):7–13.

---

prevalence of clubbing in patients with lung cancer. However, when applying bone scintigraphy changes as diagnostic criteria, the prevalence of HOA in patients with lung cancer is reduced to nearly 1%.[59]

There is no standard therapy for this syndrome. Treatment of the underlying cause remains the treatment of choice. When primary treatment is not possible, other options available include NSAIDS, analgesics, bisphosphonates, octreotide, and vagotomy.[55]

Tumor-induced Osteomalacia

Tumor-induced osteomalacia, also known as osteogenic osteomalacia, is an uncommon paraneoplastic syndrome characterized by the ectopic secretion of fibroblast growth factor 23 (FGF23).[60] Classically, this syndrome is associated with small mesenchymal tumors in which case it is called primary tumor–induced osteomalacia. Other causes have been described, including neurofibromatosis, polyostotic fibrous dysplasia, prostate cancer, oat cell cancer, and hematologic malignancies (secondary tumor–induced osteomalacia).[61]

Phosphaturic mesenchymal tumors are classified into 4 histologic variants: mixed connective tissue, osteoblastomalike, nonossifying fibromalike, and ossifying fibromalike variants. The first one is the most common, usually diagnosed as hemangiopericytoma. These tumors show positive FGF23 staining. Although they can have a benign histologic appearance, these tumors often infiltrate the surrounding tissues and in rare occasions (<5%) metastasize, mostly to the lung.[62,63] FGF23 and PTH are the major regulators of phosphate homeostasis. Physiologic actions of FGF23 include inhibition of phosphorous reabsorption on proximal tubules, downregulation of α1-hydroxylase, and upregulation of 24-hydroxylase **(Fig. 3)**.[64] Patients with tumor-induced osteomalacia present abnormal levels of serum FGF23 and develop hypophosphatemia associated with generalized weakness, multiple fractures, bone pain, and typical radiologic features of osteomalacia or rickets.[65]

Laboratory findings include hyperphosphaturia; hypophosphatemia; low or normal 1,25-dihydroxyvitamin D levels; normal serum calcium levels; high alkaline phosphatase activity; normal or high PTH levels; and, most importantly, increased serum FGF23 levels.[66]

Differential diagnoses include genetic and acquired conditions. Three genetic syndromes share a similar phenotype: X-linked hypophosphatemic rickets, autosomal

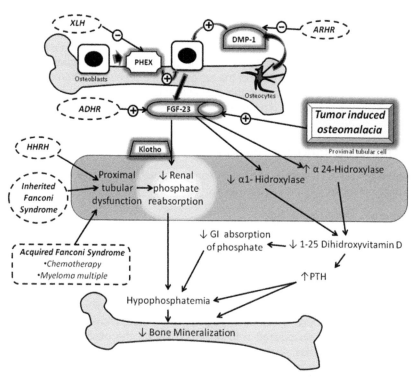

Fig. 3. Pathophysiology and differential diagnoses of tumor-induced osteomalacia. ADHR, autosomal dominant hypophosphatemic rickets; ARHR, autosomal recessive hypophosphatemic rickets; DMP1, dentin matrix acidic phosphoprotein gene; HHRH, hereditary hypophosphatemic rickets with hypercalciuria; PHEX, endopeptidases on the X chromosome gene; XLH, X-linked hypophosphatemic rickets.

dominant hypophosphatemic rickets, and autosomal recessive hypophosphatemic rickets. These syndromes are caused by mutations in FGF23 pathway, including loss of function of the phosphate-regulating gene with homologies to endopeptidases on the X chromosome protease and the dentin matrix acidic phosphoprotein 1 leading to elevated FGF23 levels that parallel the disease courses. The diagnosis is established through assessment of family history, age of onset, and genetic evaluation. Other hypophosphatemic syndromes typically have low levels of FGF23. These include hereditary hypophosphatemic rickets with hypercalciuria (also associated with nephrocalcinosis and increased 1, 25-dihydroxyvitamin D) and inherited and acquired Fanconi syndromes, which present a more extensive tubulopathy causing glucosuria, aminoaciduria, hypercalciuria, bicarbonaturia, and hypophosphatemia. FGF23 serum levels are key in differentiating tumor-induced osteomalacia, in which FGF23 level is increased, from these syndromes, in which the levels are normal or low.[60,67]

The treatment of choice for tumor-induced osteomalacia is tumor resection. Often, these tumors have very small size and are hard to find.[65] For that reason, advanced and sensitive imaging techniques are recommended first, including whole-body fludeoxyglucose F 18 PET/CT and octreotide scanning. The rationale for use of octreotide as a radiotracer is the frequent finding of somatostatin receptors in these tumors. Examples of techniques including octreotide are indium 111 octreotide single-photon emission CT and CT, and galium 68–DOTANOC (modified octreotide molecule) PET/CT. However, these techniques can lack specificity, and other techniques, such as CT and MRI, are required to confirm the diagnosis.[61] If imaging studies are not conclusive, selective venous sampling with measurement of FGF23 level is another option.[68] Despite the advances in imaging techniques, the tumor can be located only in about 60% of the cases.[61] If the precise location of the tumor is not found, medical treatment is the only available option with a therapeutic goal of maintaining a normal serum phosphorous level with phosphorous and vitamin D supplementation.[60]

IMPACT OF CANCER THERAPIES ON BONE HEALTH

Three main skeletal consequences have been associated with cancer treatment: osteoporosis, osteomalacia, and avascular necrosis.

Osteoporosis and Osteomalacia

The prevalence of osteoporosis in patients with cancer has been growing in the last decades as a direct consequence of therapeutic advances. In 2007, there were 12 million survivors of cancer in the United States, compared with 3 million in 1971.[69,70] Many of these patients are older and at increased risk for osteoporosis and fractures. There are 3 major different mechanisms that can cause osteoporosis in patients with cancer and survivors of cancer: direct bone toxicity, induced hypogonadism, and renal tubular dysfunction (**Fig. 4**).[71,72] **Table 3** shows the various therapies that have been associated with osteoporosis on the basis of the proposed mechanisms of bone loss. Among them, induction of a hypogonadal state represents the biggest impact on bone mineral density. This can occur with several different

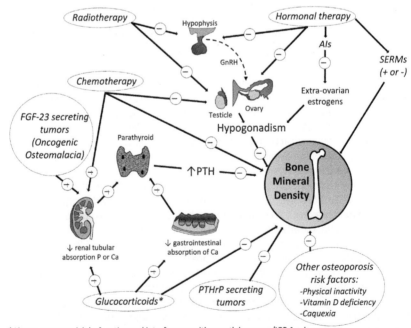

*Also causes gonadal dysfunction and interference with growth hormone/IGF-1 axis

Fig. 4. Risk factors associated with osteoporosis and osteomalacia in patients with cancer. Als, aromatase inhibitors; Ca, calcium ; GnRH, gonadotropin-releasing hormone; P, phosphorus.

Table 3
Cancer-related drugs commonly associated with osteoporosis and/or osteomalacia

Drug Group	Drug Name	Gonadal Dysfunction	Direct Bone Toxicity	Renal Tubular Dysfunction
Hormonal therapy				
SERMs	Raloxifene, Tamoxifen		✔	
AIs	Anastrazole, Letrozole, Exemestane	✔		
GnRH	Leuprolide, Goserelin	✔		
Chemotherapy				
Antimetabolite	Methotrexate		✔	
Alkylating agent	Cyclophosphamide	✔	✔	
Alkylating agent	Ifosfamide	✔		✔
Alkylating agent	Chlorambucil	✔		
Platinum	Cisplatin		?	✔
Anthracycline	Doxorubicin	✔	✔	
Tyrosine Kinase inh.	Imatinib		✔	✔
Topoisomerase II Inh.	Etoposide	✔	✔	
	Glucocorticoids	✔	✔	✔

Abbreviations: AIs, Aromatase Inhibitors; GnRH, Gonadotropin-Releasing Hormone; SERMs, Selective Estrogen Receptor Modulators.

Data from Stava CJ, Jimenez C, Hu MI, et al. Skeletal sequelae of cancer and cancer treatment. J Cancer Surviv 2009;3(2):75–88; and Fan C, Foster BK, Wallace WH, et al. Pathobiology and prevention of cancer chemotherapy-induced bone growth arrest, bone loss, and osteonecrosis. Curr Mol Med 2011;11(2):140–51.

chemotherapeutic agents as well as with hormonal therapies. Current treatment regimens for hormone-dependent cancers include hormonal drug therapy for breast and prostate cancer, oophorectomy for breast cancer, and orchiectomy for prostate cancer.[71] These patients develop rapid bone mineral loss, which results in a higher incidence of bone fractures.[73,74] Aromatase inhibitors are indicated in postmenopausal woman with estrogen receptor–positive breast cancer. These drugs inhibit estrogen production in peripheral tissues, leading to an increase in bone absorption.[75] Randomized controlled trials have shown a reduction in bone mineral density and higher incidence of bone fracture in patients receiving aromatase inhibitors versus those treated with tamoxifen.[76–82] In addition, up to 60% of patients receiving aromatase inhibitors can develop musculoskeletal symptoms, including mild to severe arthralgias, digital stiffness, carpal tunnel syndrome, and trigger fingers.[75] Selective estrogen receptor modulators (SERMs) deserve a special mention. SERMs may have agonist or antagonist effects on the bone depending on menopausal status. In premenopausal patients, their antagonist effect on circulating estrogens results in bone loss. In contrast, in postmenopausal women who have extremely low level of bioavailable estrogens, SERMs can increase bone density, lowering the risk of fractures, attributed to its estrogen agonist effect on bone.[83]

Glucocorticoids are widely used in the treatment of hematologic malignancy, prevention of chemotherapy-induced emesis for solid tumors, and treatment and prevention of graft-versus-host disease in stem cell transplant recipients. Glucocorticoids can cause rapid bone loss by directly decreasing bone formation via glucocorticoid-induced apoptosis of both osteoblasts and osteocytes and increasing bone reabsorption by prolonging the life span of preexisting osteoclasts.[84] Glucocorticoids negatively affect calcium balance by inhibiting gastrointestinal calcium absorption and renal tubular reabsorption of calcium. In addition, systemic suppressive effects of glucocorticoids on gonadal dysfunction and interference with the growth hormone/insulinlike growth factor 1 axis contribute to bone loss.[85]

Radiation therapy can also cause generalized bone loss through hypogonadism and local bone damage in the irradiated area. Radiation therapy for breast, prostate, or gynecologic cancers can lead to a higher incidence of rib or pelvic insufficiency fractures.[86,87]

Renal tubular dysfunction is another possible consequence of cancer treatment. The kidney is essential for phosphate homeostasis, and, under physiologic conditions, proximal tubules reabsorb 85% to 95% of filtered phosphate.[88] Ifosfamide, cisplatin, and imatinib are well-recognized causes of nephotoxicity.[71] These drugs damage proximal tubular cells and lead to urinary phosphate wasting. The resulting hypophosphatemia decreases bone mineralization and causes osteomalacia (see **Fig. 4**).[89] In the presence of osteomalacia, vitamin D deficiency and osteogenic osteomalacia (reviewed earlier) should also be considered. Vitamin D deficiency is the most frequent cause of osteomalacia in the general population and a well-known risk for osteoporosis and bone fractures.[90,91] High prevalence of vitamin D deficiency has been reported in patients with cancer. Napoli and colleagues[92] found a 44% prevalence of vitamin D deficiency (<20 ng/mL) and a 34% prevalence of vitamin D insufficiency (20–29 ng/mL) in patients with breast cancer. Although there is no evidence on the efficacy of vitamin D supplementation alone in reducing bone fractures in patients with cancer, higher doses of vitamin D supplementation (700–800 IU/d) have been associated with lower risk of fractures in randomized controlled trials in the general population.[90,93] Therefore, vitamin D supplementation is generally recommended in every patient with cancer at risk of bone mineral loss.[94]

Other cancer-related factors that have been associated with bone loss include physical inactivity and malnutrition.[71]

Osteonecrosis

The odds of patients with cancer developing osteonecrosis is 3.5 times higher than the general population.[95] Several cancer-related therapies have been associated with increased risk of osteonecrosis, including corticosteroids; bisphosphonates (osteonecrosis of the jaw); radiotherapy; stem cell transplantation; and, more recently reported, antiangiogenic agents (eg, sunitinib, bevacizumab).[95–100]

Corticosteroids have a direct toxic effect on bone and represent an independent risk-factor for osteonecrosis.[95] The precise mechanism is unknown but could include inhibition of bone formation and elevation of intraosseous pressure. Patients at greater risk are those receiving high doses and with other concomitant risk factors, such as having a hematopoietic malignancy, stem cell transplantation, and prior radiotheraphy.[72]

Schulte and colleagues[96] followed up 255 patients after stem cell transplantation for an observation period of at least 4 years. During this period, 11 patients developed hip osteonecrosis with a cumulative incidence of 4%. In 73% of patients, the disease was severe, and they required total hip arthroplasty. Several risk factors have been described, including higher doses of steroids, prior diagnosis other than chronic myeloid leukemia, chronic graft-versus-host disease, exposure to multiple immunosuppressant drugs, and total body irradiation.[96,98,101] It is conceivable that the development of osteonecrosis in these patients is primarily a consequence of the aggressive therapy received to treat their malignancies, induce myelosuppression, and treat graft rejection or graft-versus-host disease after the transplant.

Bisphosphonate-related osteonecrosis of the jaw occurs almost exclusively as a complication of bisphosphonate therapy in patients with cancer.[102] The true prevalence is unknown, but it has been estimated to be up to 13%.[99] Clinically this condition is defined as "the presence of exposed, necrotic bone in the oral cavity for over 6 weeks in patients with no history of radiation to the head and neck but with history of bisphosphonate use."[103] The clinical presentation can vary from mild cases with jaw pain with or without inflammatory changes on the overlying mucosa to large exposed areas of necrotic bone and osteomyelitis.[104] Osteonecrosis of the jaw has been most frequently associated with intravenous infusion of bisphosphonate for multiple myeloma, followed by metastatic breast and prostate cancer.[99] Prolonged used of intravenous nitrogen-containing bisphosphonates and history of dental problems have been recognized as the main risk factors.[102–105] In addition, zoledronic acid might be associated with a slight increased risk, with a reported osteonecrosis prevalence of 8.3% compared with 7.3% in patients exposed to pamidronate.[99] Management of osteonecrosis of the jaw can be difficult and depends on the stage and extent of the lesion. Initial treatment includes withdrawal of the inciting medication, topical rinses, systemic antibiotics, and local debridement of necrotic tissue if necessary. Advanced stages need to be referred to oral surgeons for optimal care.[104]

Patients with head and neck cancer treated with radiotherapy are also at high risk of osteonecrosis of the jaw (osteoradionecrosis). The clinical presentation and management is similar to that of osteonecrosis induced by bisphosphonates. In addition to the type of radiotherapy and total dose received, prior dental procedures are also one of the main risk factors.[97]

At present, antiangiogenic agents are found to be associated with an increased risk of osteonecrosis. In a retrospective analysis of 116 patients with cancer treated with bisphosphonates and antiangiogenic agents, 16% developed osteonecrosis of the jaw compared with 1.1% of those treated with bisphosphonates alone.[106] However, a recent analysis of 2 large randomized placebo-controlled trials evaluating bevacizumab in 1309 patients with breast cancer showed no significant difference in the incidence of osteonecrosis between the bevacizumab and placebo arms (0.3% vs 0.0%, respectively). Patients treated with additional bisphosphonates showed a higher incidence of osteonecrosis than those who were not treated (0.9% vs 0.2%), but the difference was not statistically significant.[100]

SUMMARY

Bone tumors can show a wide range of nonspecific rheumatic manifestations. The presence of unexplained or atypical chronic bone pain, an enlarging bone mass, neurovascular compression syndromes, or pathologic fractures should alert us to the possibility of a bone tumor causing these symptoms. These patients must undergo a complete physical examination; adequate imaging; and, if needed, a biopsy to confirm their diagnosis and offer them an opportune treatment.

In addition, bone tumors and other malignancies can present remote clinical manifestations and unusual laboratory findings (eg, HOA, hypophosphatemia, hyperphosphaturia, and hypercalcemia) that may be the first and early manifestation of an occult cancer. These findings should motivate a cancer screening according to age, sex, and personal history.

Cancer therapies also have a big impact on bone health, increasing the risk of osteoporosis, osteomalacia, and/or osteonecrosis. Rheumatologists should be aware of possible long-term adverse events of cancer treatment to avoid future complications.

REFERENCES

1. Wurtz LD, Peabody TD, Simon MA. Delay in the diagnosis and treatment of primary bone sarcoma of the pelvis. J Bone Joint Surg Am 1999;81(3):317–25.
2. Westhovens R, Dequeker J. Musculoskeletal manifestations of benign and malignant tumors of bone. Curr Opin Rheumatol 2003;15(1):70–5.
3. Lewis DR, Ries LAG. Cancers of the Bone and Joint. In: Ries LAG, Young JL, Keel GE, et al, editors. SEER Survival Monograph: Cancer Survival Among Adults: U.S. SEER Program, 1988-2001, Patient and Tumor Characteristics. Bethesda (MD): National Cancer Institute, SEER Program, NIH Pub. No. 07-6215; 2007. p. 81–8.
4. Jemal A, Siegel R, Xu J, et al. Cancer statistics, 2010. CA Cancer J Clin 2010; 60(5):277–300.
5. Howlader N, Noone AM, Krapcho M, et al. SEER cancer statistics review, 1975-2008. Bethesda (MD): National Cancer Institute; 2011. Available at: http://seer. cancer.gov/csr/1975_2008/. Accessed October 12, 2011. Based on 2010 SEER data submission, posted to the SEER Web site.
6. Gurney JG, Swensen AR, Bulterys M. Malignant Bone Tumors. In: Ries LAG, Smith MA, Gurney JG, et al, editors. Cancer Incidence and Survival among Children and Adolescents: United States SEER Program 1975-1995. Bethesda (MD): National Cancer Institute, SEER Program. NIH Pub. No. 99-4649; 1999. p. 99–110.
7. Coleman RE. Clinical features of metastatic bone disease and risk of skeletal morbidity. Clin Cancer Res 2006;12(20 Pt 2):6243s–9s.
8. Dubey P, Ha CS, Besa PC, et al. Localized primary malignant lymphoma of bone. Int J Radiat Oncol Biol Phys 1997;37(5):1087–93.
9. Braunstein EM. Hodgkin disease of bone: radiographic correlation with the histological classification. Radiology 1980;137(3):643–6.
10. Wyers MR. Evaluation of pediatric bone lesions. Pediatr Radiol 2010;40(4): 468–73.
11. Woertler K. Benign bone tumors and tumor-like lesions: value of cross-sectional imaging. Eur Radiol 2003;13(8):1820–35.
12. Larsson SE, Lorentzon R, Boquist L. Giant-cell tumor of bone. A demographic, clinical, and histopathological study of all cases recorded in the Swedish Cancer Registry for the years 1958 through 1968. J Bone Joint Surg Am 1975;57(2):167–73.
13. Sung HW, Kuo DP, Shu WP, et al. Giant-cell tumor of bone: analysis of two hundred and eight cases in Chinese patients. J Bone Joint Surg Am 1982; 64(5):755–61.
14. Campanacci M, Baldini N, Boriani S, et al. Giant-cell tumor of bone. J Bone Joint Surg Am 1987;69(1):106–14.
15. Viswanathan S, Jambhekar NA. Metastatic giant cell tumor of bone: are there associated factors and best treatment modalities? Clin Orthop Relat Res 2010;468(3):827–33.
16. Yildiz C, Erler K, Atesalp AS, et al. Benign bone tumors in children. Curr Opin Pediatr 2003;15(1):58–67.
17. Dorfman H, Czerniak B, Kotz R, et al. WHO classification of bone tumours. In: Fletcher C, Krishnan Unni K, Mertens F, editors. Pathology and genetics of tumours of soft tissue and bone. Lyon (France): IARCPress; 2006. p. 227–32.
18. Niembro FR, Palazuelos FI, Ortega LA. Enfermedades reumaticas, cancer y sindromes reumaticos paraneoplasicos. Mexico: McGraw-Hill Interamericana; 2007.

19. Ward WG, Eckardt JJ, Shayestehfar S, et al. Osteoid osteoma diagnosis and management with low morbidity. Clin Orthop Relat Res 1993;(291): 229–35.
20. Trapani S, Grisolia F, Simonini G, et al. Incidence of occult cancer in children presenting with musculoskeletal symptoms: a 10-year survey in a pediatric rheumatology unit. Semin Arthritis Rheum 2000;29(6):348–59.
21. Coleman RE. Skeletal complications of malignancy. Cancer 1997;80(Suppl 8): 1588–94.
22. Rud NP, Reiman HM, Pritchard DJ, et al. Extraosseous Ewing's sarcoma. A study of 42 cases. Cancer 1989;64(7):1548–53.
23. Kan P, Schmidt MH. Osteoid osteoma and osteoblastoma of the spine. Neurosurg Clin N Am 2008;19(1):65–70.
24. Perez-Martinez DA, Bueno HJ, Gutierrez F, et al. [Spinal tumors in infancy. A report of 48 cases.] Rev Neurol 1999;28(9):863–7 [in Spanish].
25. D'Angelo L, Massimi L, Narducci A, et al. Ollier disease. Childs Nerv Syst 2009; 25(6):647–53.
26. Malpas JS. Langerhans cell histiocytosis in adults. Hematol Oncol Clin North Am 1998;12(2):259–68.
27. Lietman SA, Joyce MJ. Bone sarcomas: overview of management, with a focus on surgical treatment considerations. Cleve Clin J Med 2010;77(Suppl 1): S8–12.
28. Rougraff BT. Incidental bone lesions. Instr Course Lect 2002;51:451–6.
29. Ilaslan H, Schils J, Nageotte W, et al. Clinical presentation and imaging of bone and soft-tissue sarcomas. Cleve Clin J Med 2010;77(Suppl 1):S2–7.
30. Miller TT. Bone tumors and tumorlike conditions: analysis with conventional radiography. Radiology 2008;246(3):662–74.
31. Madewell JE, Ragsdale BD, Sweet DE. Radiologic and pathologic analysis of solitary bone lesions. Part I: internal margins. Radiol Clin North Am 1981; 19(4):715–48.
32. Ragsdale BD, Madewell JE, Sweet DE. Radiologic and pathologic analysis of solitary bone lesions. Part II: periosteal reactions. Radiol Clin North Am 1981; 19(4):749–83.
33. Suva LJ, Washam C, Nicholas RW, et al. Bone metastasis: mechanisms and therapeutic opportunities. Nat Rev Endocrinol 2011;7(4):208–18.
34. Sweet DE, Madewell JE, Ragsdale BD. Radiologic and pathologic analysis of solitary bone lesions. Part III: matrix patterns. Radiol Clin North Am 1981; 19(4):785–814.
35. Mundy GR. Metastasis to bone: causes, consequences and therapeutic opportunities. Nat Rev Cancer 2002;2(8):584–93.
36. Benli IT, Akalin S, Boysan E, et al. Epidemiological, clinical and radiological aspects of osteopoikilosis. J Bone Joint Surg Br 1992;74(4):504–6.
37. Magid D. Two-dimensional and three-dimensional computed tomographic imaging in musculoskeletal tumors. Radiol Clin North Am 1993;31(2):425–47.
38. Savelli G, Maffioli L, Maccauro M, et al. Bone scintigraphy and the added value of SPECT (single photon emission tomography) in detecting skeletal lesions. Q J Nucl Med 2001;45(1):27–37.
39. Staudenherz A, Steiner B, Puig S, et al. Is there a diagnostic role for bone scanning of patients with a high pretest probability for metastatic renal cell carcinoma? Cancer 1999;85(1):153–5
40. D'Sa S, Abildgaard N, Tighe J, et al. Guidelines for the use of imaging in the management of myeloma. Br J Haematol 2007;137(1):49–63.

41. Balliu E, Boada M, Pelaez I, et al. Comparative study of whole-body MRI and bone scintigraphy for the detection of bone metastases. Clin Radiol 2010; 65(12):989–96.
42. Horger M, Bares R. The role of single-photon emission computed tomography/ computed tomography in benign and malignant bone disease. Semin Nucl Med 2006;36(4):286–94.
43. Altay M, Bayrakci K, Yildiz Y, et al. Secondary chondrosarcoma in cartilage bone tumors: report of 32 patients. J Orthop Sci 2007;12(5):415–23.
44. Schwartz HS, Zimmerman NB, Simon MA, et al. The malignant potential of enchondromatosis. J Bone Joint Surg Am 1987;69(2):269–74.
45. Strewler GJ. The physiology of parathyroid hormone-related protein. N Engl J Med 2000;342(3):177–85.
46. Burtis WJ, Brady TG, Orloff JJ, et al. Immunochemical characterization of circu-lating parathyroid hormone-related protein in patients with humoral hypercal-cemia of cancer. N Engl J Med 1990;322(16):1106–12.
47. Clines GA, Guise TA. Hypercalcaemia of malignancy and basic research on mechanisms responsible for osteolytic and osteoblastic metastasis to bone. Endocr Relat Cancer 2005;12(3):549–83.
48. Nakayama K, Fukumoto S, Takeda S, et al. Differences in bone and vitamin D metabolism between primary hyperparathyroidism and malignancy-associated hypercalcemia. J Clin Endocrinol Metab 1996;81(2):607–11.
49. Stewart AF. Clinical practice. Hypercalcemia associated with cancer. N Engl J Med 2005;352(4):373–9.
50. Wong K, Tsuda S, Mukai R, et al. Parathyroid hormone expression in a patient with metastatic nasopharyngeal rhabdomyosarcoma and hypercalcemia. Endo-crine 2005;27(1):83–6.
51. Myers KA, Farquhar DR. The rational clinical examination. Does this patient have clubbing? JAMA 2001;286(3):341–7.
52. Stavem P. Instrument for estimation of clubbing. Lancet 1959;2(7088):7–8.
53. Schamroth L. Personal experience. S Afr Med J 1976;50(9):297–300.
54. Fam AG. Paraneoplastic rheumatic syndromes. Baillieres Best Pract Res Clin Rheumatol 2000;14(3):515–33.
55. Nguyen S, Hojjati M. Review of current therapies for secondary hypertrophic pulmonary osteoarthropathy. Clin Rheumatol 2011;30(1):7–13.
56. Martinez-Lavin M. Hypertrophic osteoarthropathy. Curr Opin Rheumatol 1997; 9(1):83–6.
57. Uppal S, Diggle CP, Carr IM, et al. Mutations in 15-hydroxyprostaglandin dehy-drogenase cause primary hypertrophic osteoarthropathy. Nat Genet 2008;40(6): 789–93.
58. Sridhar KS, Lobo CF, Altman RD. Digital clubbing and lung cancer. Chest 1998; 114(6):1535–7.
59. Ito T, Goto K, Yoh K, et al. Hypertrophic pulmonary osteoarthropathy as a para-neoplastic manifestation of lung cancer. J Thorac Oncol 2010;5(7):976–80.
60. Hu MI, Yeung SCJ, Gagel RF. Endocrine paraneoplastic syndromes. In: Yeung SCJ, Escalante CP, Gagel RF, editors. Medical care of cancer patients. Shelton: People's Medical Publishing House: BC Decker Inc; 2009. p. 194–204.
61. Chong WH, Molinolo AA, Chen CC, et al. Tumor-induced osteomalacia. Endocr Relat Cancer 2011;18(3):R53–77.
62. Folpe AL, Fanburg-Smith JC, Billings SD, et al. Most osteomalacia-associated mesenchymal tumors are a single histopathologic entity: an analysis of 32

cases and a comprehensive review of the literature. Am J Surg Pathol 2004; 28(1):1–30.

63. Weidner N. Review and update: oncogenic osteomalacia-rickets. Ultrastruct Pathol 1991;15(4-5):317–33.

64. Juppner H, Wolf M, Salusky IB. FGF-23: more than a regulator of renal phosphate handling? J Bone Miner Res 2010;25(10):2091–7.

65. Farrow EG, White KE. Tumor-induced osteomalacia. Expert Rev Endocrinol Metab 2009;4(5):435–42.

66. Carpenter TO. Oncogenic osteomalacia—a complex dance of factors. N Engl J Med 2003;348(17):1705–8.

67. Halperin F, Anderson RJ, Mulder JE. Tumor-induced osteomalacia: the importance of measuring serum phosphorus levels. Nat Clin Pract Endocrinol Metab 2007;3(10):721–5.

68. Andreopoulou P, Dumitrescu CE, Kelly MH, et al. Selective venous catheterization for the localization of phosphaturic mesenchymal tumors. J Bone Miner Res 2011;26(6):1295–302.

69. Hu MI, Lu H, Gagel RF. Cancer therapies and bone health. Curr Rheumatol Rep 2010;12(3):177–85.

70. Altekruse SF, Kosary CL, Krapcho M, et al. SEER cancer statistics review, 1975–2007. Bethesda (MD): National Cancer Institute; 2010. Based on November 2009 data submission. Available at: http://seer.cancer.gov/csr/1975_2007. Accessed October 12, 2011.

71. Stava CJ, Jimenez C, Hu MI, et al. Skeletal sequelae of cancer and cancer treatment. J Cancer Surviv 2009;3(2):75–88.

72. Fan C, Foster BK, Wallace WH, et al. Pathobiology and prevention of cancer chemotherapy-induced bone growth arrest, bone loss, and osteonecrosis. Curr Mol Med 2011;11(2):140–51.

73. Chen Z, Maricic M, Bassford TL, et al. Fracture risk among breast cancer survivors: results from the Women's Health Initiative Observational Study. Arch Intern Med 2005;165(5):552–8.

74. Mittan D, Lee S, Miller E, et al. Bone loss following hypogonadism in men with prostate cancer treated with GnRH analogs. J Clin Endocrinol Metab 2002; 87(8):3656–61.

75. Gaillard S, Stearns V. Aromatase inhibitor-associated bone and musculoskeletal effects: new evidence defining etiology and strategies for management. Breast Cancer Res 2011;13(2):205.

76. Jakesz R, Jonat W, Gnant M, et al. Switching of postmenopausal women with endocrine-responsive early breast cancer to anastrozole after 2 years' adjuvant tamoxifen: combined results of ABCSG trial 8 and ARNO 95 trial. Lancet 2005; 366(9484):455–62.

77. Jakesz R, Greil R, Gnant M, et al. Extended adjuvant therapy with anastrozole among postmenopausal breast cancer patients: results from the randomized Austrian Breast and Colorectal Cancer Study Group Trial 6a. J Natl Cancer Inst 2007;99(24):1845–53.

78. Buzdar A, Howell A, Cuzick J, et al. Comprehensive side-effect profile of anastrozole and tamoxifen as adjuvant treatment for early-stage breast cancer: long-term safety analysis of the ATAC trial (Arimidex Tamoxifen Alone or in Combination Trialists' Group). Lancet Oncol 2006;7(8):633–43.

79. Forbes JF, Cuzick J, Buzdar A, et al. Effect of anastrozole and tamoxifen as adjuvant treatment for early-stage breast cancer: 100-month analysis of the ATAC

trial (Arimidex Tamoxifen Alone or in Combination Trialists' Group). Lancet Oncol 2008;9(1):45–53.

80. Coates AS, Keshaviah A, Thurlimann B, et al. Five years of letrozole compared with tamoxifen as initial adjuvant therapy for postmenopausal women with endocrine-responsive early breast cancer: update of study BIG 1-98. J Clin Oncol 2007;25(5):486–92.

81. Coombes RC, Kilburn LS, Snowdon CF, et al. Survival and safety of exemestane versus tamoxifen after 2-3 years' tamoxifen treatment (Intergroup Exemestane Study): a randomised controlled trial. Lancet 2007;369(9561):559–70.

82. Goss PE, Ingle JN, Martino S, et al. Randomized trial of letrozole following tamoxifen as extended adjuvant therapy in receptor-positive breast cancer: updated findings from NCIC CTG MA.17. J Natl Cancer Inst 2005;97(17):1262–71.

83. Vehmanen L, Elomaa I, Blomqvist C, et al. Tamoxifen treatment after adjuvant chemotherapy has opposite effects on bone mineral density in premenopausal patients depending on menstrual status. J Clin Oncol 2006;24(4):675–80.

84. Jia D, O'Brien CA, Stewart SA, et al. Glucocorticoids act directly on osteoclasts to increase their life span and reduce bone density. Endocrinology 2006; 147(12):5592–9.

85. Hochberg Z. Mechanisms of steroid impairment of growth. Horm Res 2002; 58(Suppl 1):33–8.

86. Pierce SM, Recht A, Lingos TI, et al. Long-term radiation complications following conservative surgery (CS) and radiation therapy (RT) in patients with early stage breast cancer. Int J Radiat Oncol Biol Phys 1992;23(5):915–23.

87. Igdem S, Alco G, Ercan T, et al. Insufficiency fractures after pelvic radiotherapy in patients with prostate cancer. Int J Radiat Oncol Biol Phys 2010;77(3):818–23.

88. Amanzadeh J, Reilly RF Jr. Hypophosphatemia: an evidence-based approach to its clinical consequences and management. Nat Clin Pract Nephrol 2006; 2(3):136–48.

89. Burk CD, Restaino I, Kaplan BS, et al. Ifosfamide-induced renal tubular dysfunction and rickets in children with Wilms tumor. J Pediatr 1990;117(2 Pt 1):331–5.

90. Bischoff-Ferrari HA, Willett WC, Wong JB, et al. Fracture prevention with vitamin D supplementation: a meta-analysis of randomized controlled trials. JAMA 2005; 293(18):2257–64.

91. Holick MF. Vitamin D deficiency. N Engl J Med 2007;357(3):266–81.

92. Napoli N, Vattikuti S, Ma C, et al. High prevalence of low vitamin D and musculoskeletal complaints in women with breast cancer. Breast J 2010;16(6):609–16.

93. VanderWalde A, Hurria A. Aging and osteoporosis in breast and prostate cancer. CA Cancer J Clin 2011;61(3):139–56.

94. Gralow JR, Biermann JS, Farooki A, et al. NCCN Task Force Report: bone health in cancer care. J Natl Compr Canc Netw 2009;7(Suppl 3):S1–32 [quiz: S33–5].

95. Cooper C, Steinbuch M, Stevenson R, et al. The epidemiology of osteonecrosis: findings from the GPRD and THIN databases in the UK. Osteoporos Int 2010; 21(4):569–77.

96. Schulte CM, Beelen DW. Avascular osteonecrosis after allogeneic hematopoietic stem-cell transplantation: diagnosis and gender matter. Transplantation 2004;78(7):1055–63.

97. Silvestre-Rangil J, Silvestre FJ. Clinico-therapeutic management of osteoradionecrosis: a literature review and update. Med Oral Patol Oral Cir Bucal 2011. Available at: http://www.medicinaoral.com/medoralfree01/aop/17257.pdf. Accessed October 12, 2011.

98. Fink JC, Leisenring WM, Sullivan KM, et al. Avascular necrosis following bone marrow transplantation: a case-control study. Bone 1998;22(1):67–71.
99. Migliorati CA, Woo SB, Hewson I, et al. A systematic review of bisphosphonate osteonecrosis (BON) in cancer. Support Care Cancer 2010;18(8): 1099–106.
100. Guarneri V, Miles D, Robert N, et al. Bevacizumab and osteonecrosis of the jaw: incidence and association with bisphosphonate therapy in three large prospective trials in advanced breast cancer. Breast Cancer Res Treat 2010;122(1): 181–8.
101. Campbell S, Sun CL, Kurian S, et al. Predictors of avascular necrosis of bone in long-term survivors of hematopoietic cell transplantation. Cancer 2009;115(18): 4127–35.
102. Dunstan CR, Felsenberg D, Seibel MJ. Therapy insight: the risks and benefits of bisphosphonates for the treatment of tumor-induced bone disease. Nat Clin Pract Oncol 2007;4(1):42–55.
103. Migliorati CA, Epstein JB, Abt E, et al. Osteonecrosis of the jaw and bisphosphonates in cancer: a narrative review. Nat Rev Endocrinol 2011;7(1):34–42.
104. Ruggiero SL, Dodson TB, Assael LA, et al. American Association of Oral and Maxillofacial Surgeons position paper on bisphosphonate-related osteonecrosis of the jaw— 2009 update. Aust Endod J 2009;35(3):119–30.
105. Bamias A, Kastritis E, Bamia C, et al. Osteonecrosis of the jaw in cancer after treatment with bisphosphonates: incidence and risk factors. J Clin Oncol 2005;23(34):8580–7.
106. Christodoulou CP, Pervena A, Klouvas G, et al. Combination of bisphosphonates and antiangiogenic factors induces osteonecrosis of the jaw more frequently than bisphosphonates alone. Oncology 2009;76(3):209–11.

Neoplastic and Paraneoplastic Synovitis

Maria F. Marengo, MD*, Maria E. Suarez-Almazor, MD, PhD,
Huifang Lu, MD, PhD

KEYWORDS

• Synovial tumors • Metastatic synovitis
• Paraneoplastic syndromes • Rheumatic manifestations

Arthritis can be a diagnostic challenge for clinicians because many local and systemic diseases can cause joint pain and effusion. An initial careful evaluation including a comprehensive history and physical examination is vital to establish possible differential diagnoses.[1] The patient's age, gender, and ascertainment of comorbidities, past medical and family history, and personal habits and lifestyle can provide invaluable diagnostic clues. In addition, laboratory tests on synovial fluid and imaging are often necessary to narrow down the list of possible causes.[1,2] Malignant disease often needs to be considered in the initial evaluation of patients with synovitis. Cancer can affect the synovium directly, either as a primary tumor or as a metastasis. Arthritis can also occur as a remote nonmetastatic effect of the tumor (paraneoplastic phenomenon).[3] In addition, patients with cancer receiving therapy are often immunosuppressed and therefore more susceptible to septic arthritis; they can also develop arthralgia, and sometimes synovitis, as a consequence of their treatment. This article describes the various types of arthritis that are seen in association with malignancy, and the clinical approach to the diagnosis and management of cancer-related synovitis. **Box 1** provides a list of the most frequent diseases.

PRIMARY SYNOVIAL TUMORS

Synovial lining covers joints, bursa, and tendon sheaths, and tumors can originate from any of these structures, resulting in monoarthritis or oligoarthritis, localized

Disclosures: MSA received an honorarium from Zimmer. HL received research funding from Genentech.
Section of Rheumatology, Department of General Internal Medicine, The University of Texas MD Anderson Cancer Center, 1515 Holcombe Boulevard, Unit 1465, Houston, TX 77030, USA
* Corresponding author.
E-mail address: florenciamarengo@gmail.com

Rheum Dis Clin N Am 37 (2011) 551 572
doi:10.1016/j.rdc.2011.09.008
0889-857X/11/$ – see front matter © 2011 Elsevier Inc. All rights reserved.

Box 1
Synovial tumors and cancer-related synovitis

Synovial tumors

Primary benign tumors

    Pigmented villonodular synovitis

    Synovial chondromatosis

    Hemangioma

    Lipoma arborescens

Malignant tumors

    Synovial chondrosarcoma

    Malignant pigmented villonodular synovitis

    Synovial sarcoma

Metastatic synovitis

    Adenocarcinomas

    Leukemia arthritis

    Malignant lymphoma

Paraneoplastic syndromes involving the joint

Carcinoma polyarthritis

Remitting seronegative symmetric synovitis with pitting edema

Polymyalgia rheumatica

Lupuslike syndrome

Paraneoplastic adult Still disease

Relapsing polychondritis

Jaccoud arthropathy

Amyloid arthritis

Crystal-induced arthritis

Hypertrophic osteoarthropathy

Palmar fasciitis and polyarthritis

Panniculitis and arthritis

Multicentric reticulohistiocytosis

Arthritis associated with cancer therapy

Septic arthritis

Synovitis induced by cancer therapy

Arthralgia associated with cancer therapy

---

bursitis, or single or multiple nodules. Primary synovial tumors are uncommon, and can be benign or malignant.[4,5]

Primary Benign Synovial Tumors

Of 4000 arthrotomies of the knee performed at the Mayo Clinic during a 20-year period, only 95 cases were found to have benign tumors. Among those, pigmented villonodular synovitis (PVNS) and synovial chondromatosis were the predominant diagnoses.[6]

PVNS

PVNS is a proliferative disorder of the synovial cells that leads to thickening and hypertrophy of the synovial membrane, in a villous architecture.[5] The disorder is classified as intraarticular or extraarticular according to the location, and localized or diffuse according to the pattern of growth. Intraarticular lesions often affect the knee, and may be localized or diffuse within the joint.[5,7] Localized synovitis presents as a well-defined nodule, and most frequently affects the infrapatellar fat pad of the knee. The diffuse form affects large weight-bearing joints, resulting in synovitis and sometimes a palpable mass, with serosanguinous or xanthocromic joint effusion. When the lesion originates in the tendon sheath, it is called giant cell tumor of tendon sheath. Localized lesions most commonly affect the tendons of the hand or wrist. There is a less common diffuse variant that can target tendons in the large joints of the lower extremities (diffuse giant cell tumor of tendon sheath). The diffuse variant is less well defined, with tumor projections into surrounding tissues.

PVNS was previously considered to be a reactive proliferative process; however, cytogenetic studies show clonal proliferation, consistent with a tumoral lesion.[5] Structural genetic rearrangements of 1p11 to 13 are present in both forms of PVNS. In addition, trisomies of chromosomes 5 and 7 are found, more frequently in the diffuse form. These trisomies have also been detected in malignant PVNS.[5]

Although its real incidence is unknown, PVNS is the most common benign tumor of the tendon sheaths and synovium. During a 17-year period, in a large epidemiologic study of PVNS in Memphis, Tennessee, the incidence of tenosynovitis was 9.2 cases per million per year, whereas joint synovitis alone occurred in 1.8 cases per million per year, with no bursitis reported during this period.[8] The disease is more common in women, and the mean age of the patients is 40 years.[5] A history of antecedent trauma is common, but its association with PVNS seems to be coincidental.[5]

The tumor grows slowly so the clinical onset is generally insidious, with a gradually progressive course. The clinical presentation depends on the location of the disease. It can affect any joint, but the knee is most often involved, in up to 80% of cases. Patients are often asymptomatic or can have mild pain for several years. Swelling can occur, sometimes with mechanical symptoms such as locking and catching.[7,9] Episodic joint effusions and hemarthrosis can occasionally occur and are associated with acute pain and limitation in the range of motion.[4,5] In the diffuse form, the tumor can exceed the joint, and result in locally aggressive invasion that destroys the surrounding soft tissue and bone, with progressive functional limitation at later stages. In the hands, PVNS is often situated in the lateral zone of the digit, adjacent to the interphalangeal joint, arising between the flexor and extensor tendons. The lesion is usually fixed to deep structures but is not attached to the skin. There are reports of spinal involvement, most often in the posterior elements of the cervical spine, which can cause localized pain and radicular symptoms.[10]

Radiographs may be normal or show nonspecific changes, depending on the duration of the lesion. Radiographic changes include joint effusion or increased soft tissue density, compatible with synovial hypertrophy. Erosions may be present in up to 50% of cases. Arthrography of the knee reveals localized or ill-defined filling defects, compatible with a mass or thickened synovium. Ultrasound may show joint effusion, synovial thickening, or a heterogeneous mass. Computed tomography (CT) scans can show a high-density soft tissue mass and bone lesions, but magnetic resonance imaging (MRI) is the modality of choice for diagnosis. It reveals the extent of thickening of the synovium with heterogeneous signal intensity caused by the combination of areas of low signal intensity (hemosiderin deposits and fibrous tissue) with areas of high signal intensity (fat content and congested synovium). Tumoral lesions show gadolinium enhancement. MRI is useful not only for the diagnosis but also in the preoperative planning and follow-up.[4,7,11]

A biopsy guided by CT or ultrasound may be necessary when the MRI is non-diagnostic. The histology shows villous synovial proliferation, histiocytes, foam cells, and multinucleated giant cells. The findings are consistent among the different types of lesion, except for the margins, which are well defined in localized forms but extend to adjacent tissues in the diffuse variant. Mitotic figures may be prominent, but do not show atypia. The cells tend to be arranged in clusters, separated by matrix consisting of collagen and, occasionally, osteoid and bone. Iron pigment is always present. Giant cells express an osteoclast phenotype and release proteolytic enzymes such as metalloproteinase 2 and 9, which can explain the local destructive changes. Areas of infarctlike necrosis may be found, but they are not a prominent feature.[5,12]

The treatment of PVNS is surgical. Localized disease PVNS can be successfully removed by simple excision, achieving complete relief of symptoms, with a low rate of local recurrence (<5%).[4,13]

For diffuse PVNS, a complete synovectomy is required, which can be performed arthroscopically if the lesion is confined within the joint. In cases of extraarticular involvement, open synovectomy is indicated. Incomplete synovectomy is associated with an incidence of recurrence up to 50%.[4,13] Recurrent lesions can also be a sign of malignant disease. There is evidence that low-dose postoperative radiotherapy may be beneficial in these cases.[14] Arthroplasty plus extensive synovectomy is required to avoid recurrences and in advanced cases with severe secondary osteoarthritis.[4,13]

Synovial chondromatosis

Synovial chondromatosis is a benign neoplasm of the synovial tissue, characterized by the presence of multiple metaplastic cartilaginous nodules under the surface of the synovial membrane in joints, tendons, or bursa. Osteochondromatosis, which is the ossification of these cartilaginous nodules, frequently occurs.[12] This disorder is more common in men but its true incidence is unknown. The joints most frequently affected are the knees, hips, and elbows, but unusual sites, such as the temporomandibular joint, and soft tissues around the joints, have also been reported.[15–17] No specific genetic abnormalities have been identified in association with this entity.[12,18]

Clinically, pain and synovial effusion are the most common symptoms. Locking of the joint can also occur when the cartilaginous nodules detach and become free loose bodies within the joint.[4,12] At an early stage of the disease, radiographs may be normal or only show indirect signs of swelling. Later, they can reveal typical multifocal, calcified, spherical loose bodies. Development of secondary osteoarthritis is frequent. Although CT is useful for imaging the calcifications, MRI is the preferred imaging for soft tissue assessment and it can detect chondromas at an earlier stage, when calcification has not occurred. T1-weighted images typically show multiple areas of signal void corresponding with incompletely calcified nodules. Complete cartilaginous nodules appear isointense to the muscle on T1-weighted images, whereas T2-weighted images show high signal enhancement corresponding with joint effusion and synovial proliferation.[12,19,20]

Pathologic changes include cartilaginous metaplasia of the intimal layer in a solid matrix without myxoid change. Calcification between chondrocytes is common.[12,20]

Treatment consists of the surgical removal of loose bodies by arthroscopy or synovectomy. Recurrence can occur in approximately 30% of cases. Secondary osteoarthritis is frequent, but malignant transformation is extremely rare.[4,17–19]

Synovial hemangioma

Synovial hemangioma is a rare benign vascular tumor of the synovium. The knee is most commonly affected, followed by the shoulder and the ankle.[4,12] It typically occurs in adolescents who report a history of pain in the affected joint and can develop recurrent atraumatic hemartrosis.[21–23] Radiographs are normal or show nonspecific features. MRI is the preferred imaging modality for diagnosis, although angiography also accurately shows vascular lesions. Histologically, there is proliferation of vessels, capillary or cavernous, in the synovium.[12] Preoperative embolization can be useful.[24,25] Treatment involves the complete surgical removal of the involved area.[4,5,12]

Lipoma arborescens

Lipoma arborescens is a benign lipomatous proliferation involving the synovium.[4] This condition is rare, and occurs most frequently in men in the fourth and fifth decades of life. The knee is most commonly affected.[4,12] Symptoms include joint effusion and locking. MRI reveals characteristic villous synovial masses with enhanced fat intensity signal.[4,5,26] Histologically, the lesion consists of typical mature fatty tissue in the subsynovium.[12] Treatment consists of the complete removal of involved synovium. Recurrence is rare.[12,18]

Primary Malignant Synovial Tumors

Synovial chondrosarcoma

This malignant neoplasia of the hyaline cartilage can originate from existing synovial chondromatosis or develop de novo.[12] It is extremely rare, with only a few cases reported.[27–32] There is a female predominance, and the age at onset ranges between 30 and 70 years.

Clinical presentation resembles the characteristics of the benign variant, but the progression is faster.[33] MRI shows findings similar to those of synovial chondromatosis; however, the mass is larger and the bone is usually compromised.[33] The biopsy shows cartilaginous nodules, but chondrocytes have a sheetlike arrangement and the matrix shows marked myxoid changes. Cellular atypia is moderate, with spindle cells surrounding the nodules; the adjacent bone may be infiltrated.[5,12]

If complete removal is successful, recurrence is rare. However, this is often difficult to achieve, and the overall prognosis is poor, with a mortality of up to 50%.[34]

Malignant PVNS

Malignant PVNS (MPVNS) is extremely rare and it can be difficult to differentiate from benign aggressive PVNS. It is unclear whether this malignancy arises de novo or in areas of benign PVNS. Some investigators reserve this diagnosis for lesions in which a typical-appearing benign PVNS coexists with frankly malignant areas, or when the original lesion is typical of a benign variant and the recurrence seems to be malignant.[5] Swelling and pain of the affected joint are the main symptoms.[12,35,36]

Biopsy reveals nodules that invade surrounding soft tissues, with diffuse, compact sheets and fascicles of oval and round cells with large hyperchromatic nuclei and more prominent nucleoli than are found in typical cases of PVNS. Atypical mitosis is seen, as well as diffuse necrotic areas.[5,37]

Wide excision is essential to avoid recurrences, and amputation is required in some cases. These patients require long-term follow-up for local recurrence or metastatic disease even years after the initial presentation.[5,38] Prognosis is not well documented; a case series reported by Bertoni and colleagues[37] showed a mortality of 50% associated with pulmonary metastases.

Synovial sarcoma

Synovial sarcoma includes a spectrum of uncommon mesenchymal neoplasms that histologically resemble synovium, but there is not sufficient evidence that it truly arises from, or differentiates into, synovium.[5] In general, the tumor develops primarily from soft tissues in periarticular regions of the extremities, usually the legs, and then invades the joint. Primary synovial sarcoma originating from articular synovium is extremely rare.

Synovial sarcoma accounts for 6% of all soft tissue sarcomas, with an incidence of 2.75 per 100,000 per year. It affects young adults 15 to 40 years of age, most commonly men.[5] The most common manifestation is a painless mass, which occurred in half of the patients in one study.[39] Less frequently, pain can be the initial complaint (15%). The presence of constitutional symptoms is rare (2%).[39,40]

Radiographic findings show a round or oval radiopacity, usually located in close proximity to a large joint. About 20% of cases present a periosteal reaction or involvement of the underlying bone. The most characteristic radiologic finding is the presence of multiple spotty calcifications, found in 15% to 20% of patients. CT does not provide additional specific findings and MRI is useful for determining the extent of the lesion.[5,41]

Two types of histology have been recognized. The classic biphasic type consists of epithelial cells lining glandular spaces that secrete chondroitin sulfate and hyaluronic acid, surrounded by fibroblastlike spindle cells that also secrete mucinous material. The monophasic variety is found in 39% of all cases, and only contains spindle cells arranged in cords, sheets, or nests.[5,12,39]

Almost all patients present specific genetic translocations [t(X;18)(p11.2;q11.2)] that are rarely associated with other types of sarcomas. The translocation involves the fusion of the SYT gene on chromosome 18 with either the SSX1 or SSX2 gene on the X chromosome.[5] Most tumors with SYT-SSX2 are monophasic, whereas almost all biphasic tumors have the SYT-SSX1 fusion.[12,42,43]

In general, the tumor grows slowly, with a well-defined appearance, giving a misleading impression of a benign process that can delay the diagnosis for years. Metastatic lesions develop in about 50% of cases, most commonly to the lung, bone, and regional lymph nodes.[5] Factors associated with poor prognosis include large tumor size, invasion of bone and neurovascular structures, metastases at the time of diagnosis, high-grade histology, and insufficient surgical resection. Treatment requires wide local resection or amputation.[5] Recent evidence shows favorable oncologic and functional outcomes with wide excision surgery along with plastic surgery reconstruction to facilitate limb salvage.[44] Surgery is often followed by radiation or chemotherapy. A recent study suggested that synovial sarcomas are more responsive to doxorubicin and ifosfamide treatment than other soft tissue sarcomas.[45]

Local recurrence after adequate treatment is about 40%. Patients with synovial sarcoma should be followed for more than 10 years because of the high risk of developing late metastases with high mortality.[46] Reported 5-year survival rates for synovial sarcoma range from 36% to 76%, and only 20% to 63% live for more than 10 years.[5] Synovial sarcomas have immunohistochemical overexpression of the epidermal growth factor receptor (EGFR), and new targeted treatment options have emerged recently, using EGFR antagonists.[47]

METASTATIC SYNOVITIS
Solid Tumors

Arthritis caused by metastatic synovitis is a rare manifestation of solid tumors. Typically, there is a monoarthritis of a large joint, the knee being most frequently involved (>50%), commonly with a metastasis in the adjacent bone. There are many reported cases in the literature, most of them usually associated with adenocarcinoma, especially bronchogenic carcinoma and, less frequently, colon, renal cell, laryngeal, and breast carcinoma.[48–51] Synovial fluid in malignant joint disease is usually sanguineous and noninflammatory. Cytologic examination of the synovial fluid can detect atypical cells (45%–63%), avoiding the need for biopsy of the synovium.[51,52] Radiographs can be normal or show a lesion in the adjacent bone when it is compromised, which can also show increased uptake in technetium-99 bone scans.[51] It is important to consider a synovial metastasis in patients with a history of previous malignancy presenting with unexplained monoarthritis, especially of a large joint. Generally, prognosis is poor, with average survival of less than 5 months.[51] In addition to treatment of the underlying malignancy, palliative treatment with chemotherapy or radiation therapy in the affected joint usually provides relief of symptoms.[51]

Leukemic Arthritis

Leukemic arthritis needs to be suspected in patients with leukemia who develop unexplained joint pain and swelling.[53] The overall prevalence of leukemic arthritis in patients with leukemia is estimated to be 4% in adults and 14% in children.[53] It is more frequent in acute than in chronic leukemia, and it can occur at any time in the course of the disease. Several mechanisms have been described, including direct infiltration of leukemic cells into the synovium, synovial reaction to periosteal or capsular infiltration, and hemorrhage caused by thrombocytopenia. Immune complex disease has also been proposed as a cause of arthritis in these patients. Overall, the predominant mechanism seems to be synovial infiltration.[53] The arthritis is most commonly asymmetric and oligoarticular, and the joint most frequently affected is the knee. Typically, the patient complains of severe pain, out of proportion to the degree of the joint effusion, and often accompanied by systemic fever. Analysis of the synovial fluid is not always helpful, because blast cells are not commonly found in the synovial fluid. Blinded synovial biopsies may miss a focus of leukemic cells. Immunofluorescence, immunocytologic analyses, and flow cytometry are techniques that allow an increased diagnostic yield. Symptomatic treatment is disappointing. Leukemic arthritis improves with successful treatment of the underlying disease; refractory cases can be treated with radiation therapy.[53,54]

Malignant Lymphomas

Lymphoma infiltration of the joints is extremely rare. In a series of more than 37,000 cases of lymphoma during a 6-year period, Krüger and colleagues[55] reported only 20 cases (0.05%) of secondary infiltration of the joint. Large joints were more affected and low-grade lymphomas were more prevalent. Survival time was variable, ranging between 11 and 27 months, depending on the grade of malignancy and tumoral extension.[55]

PARANEOPLASTIC SYNOVITIS

Paraneoplastic syndromes are a group of heterogeneous disorders associated with malignant diseases but that are not directly caused by the physical effects of the primary tumor or its metastases. The syndromes may be caused by (1) tumor production of substances that directly or indirectly cause distant symptoms; (2) depletion of normal substances, leading to paraneoplastic manifestation; or (3) host response to the tumor that results in the syndrome.[56] The paraneoplastic syndrome may precede, coexist with, or develop after the cancer is diagnosed. It usually follows a parallel course with the tumor, generally improves, and even remits with the treatment of the underlying disease, and relapses with recurrences.

A patient with a malignant disease can present various rheumatic manifestations such as arthralgia, arthritis, myositis, vasculitis, panniculitis, or fasciitis. It is necessary to determine whether these manifestations are related to the malignancy, or whether they represent a primary rheumatic disease or adverse events associated with drug therapies. Clinicians should be aware of a paraneoplastic syndrome as the first sign of an occult malignancy, and its recognition may be critical for early tumor detection.[57] This article reviews those rheumatic paraneoplastic syndromes that can present with synovitis.

Many paraneoplastic syndromes causing synovitis have been described in the literature. All of them are rare and epidemiologic evidence is scarce. The literature mostly consists of case reports and series that are insufficient to establish true prevalence or incidence rates.

Carcinoma Polyarthritis

This syndrome occurs in older patients with cancer and is characterized by abrupt onset of asymmetric arthritis, which can be oligoarticular or polyarticular, and with a migratory or additive pattern. It most often involves the large joints of the lower extremities, sparing the joints of the hands. Generally, the synovitis is not associated with erosions, deformities, or rheumatoid nodules, and previous family history of rheumatoid arthritis and rheumatoid factor are negative.[58] However, symmetric arthritis, resembling rheumatoid arthritis, has been reported.[59,60] In a series of 13 patients, rheumatoid factor was detected in 46%.[58] This finding could be explained by the underlying malignancy and older age of patients, which can be associated with positive rheumatoid factor.[3,58] The use of the anticyclic citrullinated peptide (anti-CCP) could be useful in these cases because the test seems to be negative in cancer-related arthritis.[61–64]

The synovial fluid can be mildly inflammatory and the biopsy shows nonspecific synovitis. The differential diagnosis for carcinoma polyarthritis is broad and it is often a diagnosis of exclusion.[58] Because it occurs in patients with advanced age, one of the most important differential disorders is late-onset rheumatoid arthritis, which can be difficult to exclude because carcinoma polyarthritis can appear before the diagnosis of cancer.

Carcinoma polyarthritis occurs in association with solid tumors such as breast, colon, lung, gastric, and ovarian cancer, as well as lymphoproliferative disorders.[3,58] The pathogenesis of the disorder has not been clearly elucidated. Possible mechanisms include the deposit of immune complexes in the synovium, and cross reactivity between tumor antigens and the synovium. The arthritis usually responds to nonsteroidal antiinflammatory drugs (NSAIDs) and steroids. Its course can follow the underlying disease, with remissions depending on the response of the tumor to cancer therapy.[3,65]

Remitting Seronegative Symmetric Synovitis with Pitting Edema

The syndrome of remitting seronegative symmetric synovitis with pitting edema (RS3PE) may be the initial manifestation of an idiopathic rheumatic disease in elderly patients or may present as a paraneoplastic condition. It is characterized by the sudden onset of symmetric arthritis involving predominantly the wrists, carpal joints, small hand joints, and the flexor sheaths, accompanied by marked dorsal swelling of the hands with pitting edema (boxing-glove hand). Pitting edema over the feet and pretibial areas is also observed in some patients. Typically, acute-phase reactants are increased, rheumatoid factor is persistently seronegative, and the edema is sensitive to small doses of steroids.[66]

Paraneoplastic RS3PE is associated with several solid and hematologic malignancies. Prostatic, colonic, gastric, ovarian, and endometrial adenocarcinomas are the most commonly associated solid tumors.[67,68] RS3PE has also been reported in patients with chronic lymphocytic leukemia, lymphoma, and myelodysplastic syndrome. The pathogenic mechanism is unknown but it has been postulated that the underlying neoplasia induces an immunogenic T cell inflammatory response.[69] The presence of systemic signs and symptoms such as fever, anorexia, and weight loss, and poor response to low doses of steroids (10 mg/d), suggest paraneoplastic RS3PE.[67]

Polymyalgia Rheumatica

Polymyalgia rheumatica is an inflammatory rheumatic condition in elderly patients, characterized by aching and morning stiffness in the truncal and proximal muscle groups of the shoulder, hip girdle, and neck area. In addition, it can be associated with an asymmetric and nonerosive synovitis, which usually affects knees, wrists, and metacarpophalangeal joints. Its association with malignancy is controversial, as are the recommendations for potential investigation of coexistent malignancy.[70,71] Naschitz[71,72] summarized atypical features of polymyalgia rheumatica that could suggest underlying occult cancer: age less than 50 years, asymmetric involvement, erythrocyte sedimentation rate less than 40 or higher than 100 mm/h, poor response to low doses of steroids, and long-lasting symptoms. Hematologic malignancies have been more frequently associated with this disorder, although solid tumors have also been reported recently.[73]

Lupuslike Syndrome

This syndrome resembles systemic lupus erythematosus, and is characterized by nondeforming arthritis, serositis and Raynaud phenomenon. Antinuclear antibody is positive in 70% and anti–double-stranded deoxyribonucleic acid (DNA) in 50% of the cases. It has been associated with breast, lung and ovarian cancer, leukemia, and lymphoma.[74–79] Treatment consists of NSAIDs and steroids.

Paraneoplastic Adult Still Disease

Adult Still disease is manifested by polyarthralgias/arthritis, spiking fever, and evanescent macular erythematous eruption. The association between this condition and cancer is uncommon and uncertain, and only a few cases have been reported in the literature.[80–82]

Relapsing Polychondritis

Relapsing polychondritis is a rare disorder, diagnosed if at least 3 of the following signs are present: bilateral chondritis of the external ears, inflammatory polyarthritis, ocular inflammation, nasal chondritis, vestibular/auditory malfunction, and respiratory tract chondritis.[83] A few cases have been described in association with malignancies, but causality remains uncertain.[84–87] Symptomatic treatment consists of NSAIDs or steroids.[83]

Jaccoud Arthropathy

Jaccoud arthropathy is a rapidly developing, nonerosive, deforming arthropathy, most commonly affecting the hands. On physical examination, no true joint effusion or tenderness is found, and there is no synovitis. It has been reported as the initial manifestation of lung carcinoma, but its causal relationship with cancer at large remains unclear.[88]

Amyloid Arthritis

Amyloid arthropathy occurs in patients with multiple myeloma and results from the deposition of monoclonal light chains in the synovium. In a series of 43 patients with multiple myeloma, only 2 had amyloid arthritis.[89] This synovitis can resemble rheumatoid arthritis with symmetric involvement of the upper extremities involving shoulders, wrists, and the small joints of the hands. The typical shoulder-pad sign is a visible enlargement of the anterior shoulder that results from swelling of the glenohumeral joint and amyloid deposition in periarticular soft tissues. Arthrocentesis reveals a noninflammatory synovial fluid and the sediment contains amyloid bodies that are synovial villi with amyloid deposits. Under polarized light microscopy using Congo Red staining, the amyloid deposits in the synovium and in the sediment appear apple-green birefringent. The presence of other clinical manifestations, including peripheral neuropathy, carpal tunnel syndrome, macroglossia, cardiomyopathy, and nephropathy, should alert the clinician to this potential diagnosis.[89,90]

Therapy primarily consists of treating the underlying myeloma, and symptomatic treatment with analgesic or NSAIDs. The prognosis is poor.[89]

Crystal-Induced Arthritis

Although gout and pseudogout are not always included in the classification of paraneoplastic arthritis, they can be considered as such because they can be caused by a substance, uric acid, produced through tumor lysis and resulting in remote effects such as gouty arthritis or, in severe cases, tumor lysis syndrome. The diagnosis is confirmed by the presence of crystals and inflammatory exudate in the synovial fluid.[91] Secondary gout can occur with malignancies in which hyperuricemia is frequent through (1) increased urate production, as seen in myeloproliferative and lymphoproliferative disorders, and in solid tumors with the use of cytotoxic chemotherapy[92]; and (2) decreased renal clearance induced by drugs such as cyclosporine and tacrolimus.[91] Although hyperuricemia is frequent in patients who have cancer, it is unclear how often these patients develop gouty arthritis. In a series of 63 patients with myeloproliferative disorders and gout, the development of arthritis was associated with the duration of the hematologic illness. In comparison with primary gout, patients with tumor-related gouty arthritis tend to be older, have no family history of gout, and have a higher prevalence of nephrolithiasis and tophi. Typical podagra is not common, with knees, elbows, and ankles being the most frequently affected joints. Generally, this arthritis is less responsive to routine therapy than primary gout.[93] Preventive measures include aggressive intravenous hydration and the administration of hypouricemic agents, such as allopurinol, febuxostat, or rasburicase.[94]

Pseudogout is caused by intraarticular deposition of calcium pyrophosphate dehydrate (CPPD) crystals. It most often occurs as monoarthritis or oligoarthritis. Plain radiographs show stippled calcifications of articular and meniscal cartilage (chondrocalcinosis) predominantly in knees, wrists, hips, and the pubic symphysis.[95] Pseudogout can occur in patients who have cancer who develop severe and persistent hypercalcemia. This hypercalcemia can be caused by the ectopic secretion of different substances (PTH-related protein, 1,25-$(OH)_2D_3$, or cytokines) by the tumor. Hypercalcemia is most commonly observed in patients with lung, breast, and hematologic cancer.[96] The increased serum calcium may predispose to CPPD crystallization in the joint.[97] Joint aspiration combined with steroid injection is often sufficient for acute CPPD arthritis. In recurrent cases, oral NSAIDs and/or low-dose colchicine may relieve the symptoms. Low-dose corticosteroids, methotrexate, and hydroxychloroquine have been used in patients with primary chronic disease unresponsive to other therapies.[98]

Hypertrophic Osteoarthropathy

Hypertrophic osteoarthropathy (HOA) is a syndrome characterized by abnormal proliferation of the skin and osseous tissue at the distal parts of the extremities. Prominent clinical features of HOA include digital clubbing and periostitis of tubular bones. Mild accompanying synovitis can also occur, most commonly in the knees, ankles, wrists, and metacarpophalangeal joints. The synovial fluid is a noninflammatory liquid, however the histology shows mild synovitis with vascular dilatation and sparse lymphocytic infiltration.[99,100]

Plain radiographs reveal periosteal thickening that can involve only a few bones or all tubular bones, with normal joints. Acro-osteolysis may be found in severe and long-standing cases. Isotopic bone scans can show a pericortical, linear concentration of the radionuclide along the shafts of affected bones and allow detection in early stages, even before the development of symptoms.[101,102]

HOA is most often associated with non–small cell lung cancer (squamous cell or adenocarcinoma). Other rarely associated tumors include nasopharyngeal cancer, mesothelioma, renal cell carcinoma, esophageal cancer, gastric tumor, pancreatic cancer, breast phyllodes tumor, melanoma, thymic cancer, and Hodgkin lymphoma.[103–106]

The pathogenesis remains unknown and several theories have been proposed. Initially, neural involvement was thought to play a role, given the good response to vagotomy and atropine.[107,108] More recently, it has been observed that platelet-derived growth factors (PDGF) are increased in HOA, and some investigators have proposed that the release of PDGF-like factors by neoplasia can cause this disorder.[109]

If the primary cause can be treated, the symptoms of HOA are most likely to improve or resolve. Symptomatic treatment includes analgesics, NSAIDs, or low-dose steroids, if needed. Unilateral thoracic vagotomy has been used in the past for severe cases in patients with lung cancer. Bisphosphonates and somatostatin analogues such as octreotide have also been proposed as therapy.[110–113]

Palmar Fasciitis and Polyarthritis

Palmar fasciitis is a disabling paraneoplastic condition characterized by a severe symmetric thickening of the palmar fascia affecting the flexor retinaculum and the flexor tendons of the hands, resulting in claw hands. Articular involvement of the upper extremities can occur, and, in the shoulders, it can result in severe adhesive capsulitis. The course of the disease is severe and rapidly progressive.[114]

This fibrosing disorder was initially described in patients with ovarian carcinoma.[115] More recently, it has also been associated with breast, lung, pancreatic, stomach, prostate, and uterine cancer.[116–118] Clinical differential diagnoses include Dupuytron, scleroderma, eosinophilic fasciitis, reflex sympathetic dystrophy, and diabetic cheiroarthropathy.

Treatment is disappointing. The symptoms rarely respond to analgesics, NSAIDs, steroids, physical therapy, or ganglion blockade. In general, successful tumoral excision is followed by an improvement of the symptoms, or at least by the arrest of the progression.[116–118]

Panniculitis and Arthritis

Paraneoplastic panniculitis results from subcutaneous fat necrosis with the subsequent development of multiple erythematous and painful nodules, often in the lower extremities. The nodules may ulcerate and secrete an oily substance. When they develop adjacent to a joint, a reactive synovitis can occur. Skin biopsy shows steatonecrosis, and ghost-like cells characterized by a thick wall with no nucleus are pathognomonic of this condition.[114,119,120]

This entity is associated with pancreatitis and pancreatic cancer, and should be suspected in patients who present with weight loss and jaundice.[121] However, it usually occurs late in the course of the disease and may not be helpful for an early diagnosis of pancreatic cancer.[115] It has been postulated that the lipase and amylase that are increased in the serum of these patients increase the permeability of the microcirculation, inducing fat necrosis.[122] Treatment is challenging because panniculitis is often resistant to treatment with steroids.[3]

Multicentric Reticulohistiocytosis

Multicentric reticulohistiocytosis is a systemic disease of unknown cause, characterized by a reactive proliferation of histiocytes in nodules in the skin, mucosa, subcutaneous tissue, synovium, and bone. This disorder is very rare, and a review of 96 case reports published in the last 34 years describes an association with cancer in up to 31%.[123] Articular involvement is the initial manifestation in 40% of the patients, associated with skin lesions in 29%.[123] The arthritis most often affects the wrists, metacarpophalangeal joints, and distal interphalangeal joints, although any joint can be involved. Typically, the arthritis is destructive with radiographic marginal erosions. The clinical course can be relapsing and remitting, and can be severe with progression to arthritis mutilans.[123,124]

Skin lesions show reddish, brown, pink, or gray papules or nodules that typically affect hands, face, trunk, legs, and mucosa. These lesions can cluster around the nail, resulting in an appearance of a string of coral beads, which is pathognomonic. In addition, xanthelasmas and vermicular lesions bordering the nostrils are found.[124] Skin biopsy shows histiocytic multinucleated giant cells with eosinophilic, finely granulated, and ground-glass cytoplasm, which are hallmarks of the disease.[123]

Treatment consists of analgesics, NSAIDs, and steroids as needed. Successful treatment has been reported using alkylating agents,[125] methotrexate,[126] and, more recently, with tumor necrosis factor inhibitors.[127,128] This paraneoplastic disorder can persist despite treatment of the concomitant malignancy. Nevertheless, it usually remits spontaneously after a few years.[124]

ARTHRITIS ASSOCIATED WITH CANCER THERAPY
Septic Arthritis

Compared with the general population, patients with cancer have additional risk factors that predispose them to infections. These risk factors include impaired host defenses by the malignancy itself, the drugs used to treat it, the use of long-standing venous catheters, and frequent hospitalizations.[129]

Septic arthritis usually results from hematogenous spread from another site of infection. The most common infectious agent is *Staphylococcus aureus*, originated from infections related to wounds, decubitus ulcers, or long-term use of central venous catheter.[130] In addition, unusual presentations have been reported with certain malignancies. Septic arthritis caused by unusual enteric pathogens, such as group G *Streptococcus* and *Clostridium septicum* can occur in patients with colonic cancer.[131–133] Pyogenic arthritis of the shoulder has also been reported after treatment of ipsilateral breast cancer.[3]

Although bacteria are the most common cause of septic arthritis, clinicians should be alert to the possibility of infection by less common pathogens in this immunocompromised population.[1] Clinically, the onset of mycobacterial and fungal arthritis is insidious and the course is indolent, which can delay diagnosis and treatment.[134,135] Currently, because of the widespread use of fungal prophylaxis with fluconazole, the incidence of *Candida albicans* has been reduced in patients with hematologic diseases. However, non–*C albicans* species that have natural resistance to fluconazole have emerged as new fungal pathogens.[136] Other *Candida* strains recently reported are *Candida tropicalis* and *Candida krusei*, with most of the cases occurring in neutropenia with hematologic malignancies.[137–142]

The diagnosis of septic arthritis is a clinical emergency. Treatment requires appropriate antimicrobials, along with joint drainage.

Arthritis Associated with Cancer Therapy

Many drugs or procedures used to treat cancer can induce synovitis. Interferon-α is used for the treatment of lymphoma and carcinoid tumors and has been associated with the development of autoimmune syndromes that can clinically resemble rheumatoid arthritis, polymyositis, or systemic lupus erythematosus.[143,144]

There are other unusual reported cases of arthritis associated with cancer therapy. Autologous stem cell transplantation for lymphoid malignancies has been associated with the development of spondyloarthropathy in patients positive for human leukocyte antigen B27.[145] Bacille Calmette-Guérin immunotherapy used for the treatment of superficial bladder carcinoma can also cause a reactive polyarthritis.[146]

Unlike true arthritis caused by cancer therapy, which is very rare, arthralgia is common in this setting. Aromatase inhibitors are compounds that inhibit aromatase to reduce the production of estrogenic steroid hormones in postmenopausal women. They are used for treating early stage hormone-receptor-positive breast cancer. Aromatase inhibitors are associated with arthralgia in up to 47% of women with breast cancer receiving these agents.[147] True joint damage is not observed, but many patients discontinue therapy because of persistent joint symptoms that impair their quality of life.

Postchemotherapy rheumatism is a self-limited, migratory, noninflammatory arthropathy that has been described with different drugs including cyclophosphamide, 5-fluorouracil, methotrexate, and tamoxifen. Symptoms appear after several weeks or months following the treatment and usually remit within weeks or months after completion of treatment.[148] Taxanes (paclitaxel and docetaxel) can also cause severe pain in muscles and joints, but the symptoms typically begin 1 or 2 days after the infusion and last for a median of 4 to 5 days.[149]

SUMMARY

Arthritis is a common finding in patients who have cancer. In this population, it is crucial to rule out septic arthritis and metastatic synovitis. Culture, crystallography,

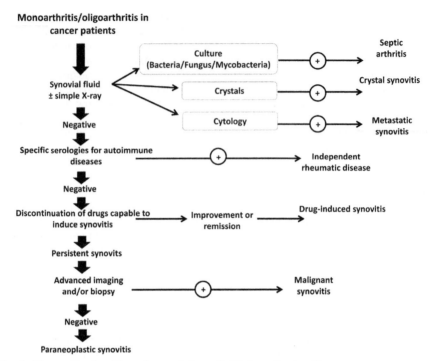

Fig. 1. Diagnostic algorithm of mono/oligoarthritis in patients with cancer.

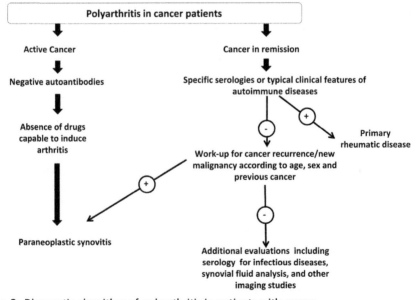

Fig. 2. Diagnostic algorithm of polyarthritis in patients with cancer.

and cytology of synovial fluid are useful initial diagnostics tools. If all are negative, histopathology of synovial tissue should be considered (**Figs. 1** and **2**).

Crystal synovitis is another frequent cause of arthritis in patients who have cancer, but it can also coexist with other conditions such as septic arthritis. Independent rheumatic disorders, drug-induced arthritis, and paraneoplastic syndromes should be considered after the exclusion of sepsis and metastatic disease. The diagnosis of a paraneoplastic syndrome is easier when the malignancy is evident or typical findings such as HOA or palmar fasciitis are present. However, these paraneoplastic phenomena can occur before the cancer diagnosis, and it is important to be aware of the association of these conditions with an underlying tumor. Rheumatic disorders with atypical clinical presentation in older patients, poor response to usual treatment, systemic features such as weight loss, and clinical findings compatible with well-recognized paraneoplastic syndromes should alert clinicians to the possible coexistence of an occult malignancy.

ACKNOWLEDGMENTS

The authors would like to acknowledge the contribution of Greg Pratt, who assisted us with the bibliography.

REFERENCES

1. Sack K. Monarthritis: differential diagnosis. Am J Med 1997;102(1A):30S–4S.
2. Ma L, Cranney A, Holroyd-Leduc JM. Acute monoarthritis: what is the cause of my patient's painful swollen joint? CMAJ 2009;180(1):59–65.
3. Fam AG. Paraneoplastic rheumatic syndromes. Baillieres Best Pract Res Clin Rheumatol 2000;14(3):515–33.
4. Adelani MA, Wupperman RM, Holt GE. Benign synovial disorders. J Am Acad Orthop Surg 2008;16(5):268–75.
5. Weiss S, Goldblum J. Enziger and Weiss's soft tissue tumours. 5th edition. Philadelphia (PA): Mosby/Elsevier; 2008.
6. Coventry MB, Harrison EG, Martin JF. Benign synovial tumors of the knee: a diagnostic problem. J Bone Joint Surg Am 1966;48(7):1350–8.
7. Kransdorf M, Murphey M. Imaging of soft tissue tumors. 2nd edition. Philadelphia (PA): Lippincott Williams & Wilkins; 2006.
8. Myers B, Masi A. Pigmented villonodular synovitis and tenosynovitis: a clinical epidemiologic study of 166 cases and literature review. Medicine (Baltimore) 1980;59(3):223–38.
9. Rao S, Rae P, Royle S, et al. Localized pigmented villonodular synovitis presenting as a locked knee: a report of three cases and a review of the literature. Knee 1995;2(3):173–6.
10. Furlong MA, Motamedi K, Laskin WB, et al. Synovial-type giant cell tumors of the vertebral column: a clinicopathologic study of 15 cases, with a review of the literature and discussion of the differential diagnosis. Hum Pathol 2003;34(7):670–9.
11. Al-Nakshabandi N, Ryan AG, Choudur H, et al. Pigmented villonodular synovitis. Clin Radiol 2004;59:414–20.
12. Unni KK, Inwards CY, Bridge JA, et al. Tumors of the bones and joints. AFIP atlas of tumor pathology. Washington, DC: American registry of pathology in collaboration with the Armed Forces Institute of pathology; Bethesda, (MD): ARP Press; 2005.
13. Otluoglu O. Pigmented villonodular synovitis. Orthop Clin North Am 2006;37: 23–33.

14. Berger B, Ganswindt U, Bamberg M, et al. External beam radiotherapy as post-operative treatment of diffuse pigmented villonodular synovitis. Int J Radiat Oncol Biol Phys 2007;67(4):1130–4.

15. Miyamoto H, Sakashita H, Wilson DF, et al. Synovial chondromatosis of the temporomandibular joint. Br J Oral Maxillofac Surg 2000;38(3):205–8.

16. Ronald JB, Keller EE, Weiland LH. Synovial chondromatosis of the temporomandibular joint. J Oral Surg 1978;36(1):13–9.

17. Coles MJ, Tara HH Jr. Synovial chondromatosis: a case study and brief review. Am J Orthop (Belle Mead NJ) 1997;26(1):37–40.

18. Szendroi M, Deodhar A. Synovial neoformations and tumours. Best Pract Res Clin Rheumatol 2000;14(2):363–83.

19. Conrad E. Orthopaedic oncology: diagnosis and treatment. New York: Thieme Medical Publishers; 2009.

20. Beall DP, Ly JQ, Wolff JD, et al. Cystic masses of the knee: magnetic resonance imaging findings. Curr Probl Diagn Radiol 2005;34(4):143.

21. Hawley WL, Ansell BM. Synovial haemangioma presenting as monarticular arthritis of the knee. Arch Dis Child 1981;56(7):558–60.

22. Rajni, Khanna G, Gupta A, et al. Synovial hemangioma: a rare benign synovial lesion. Indian J Pathol Microbiol 2008;51(2):257–8.

23. Winzenberg T, Ma D, Taplin P, et al. Synovial haemangioma of the knee: a case report. Clin Rheumatol 2006;25(5):753–5.

24. Akgun I, Kesmezacar H, Ogut T, et al. Intra-articular hemangioma of the knee. Arthroscopy 2003;19(3):E17.

25. Vakil-Adli A, Zandieh S, Hochreiter J, et al. Synovial hemangioma of the knee joint in a 12-year-old boy: A case report. J Med Case Reports 2010; 4:105.

26. Martin S, Hernandez L, Romero J, et al. Diagnostic imaging of lipoma arborescens. Skeletal Radiol 1998;27(6):325–9.

27. Hallam P, Ashwood N, Cobb J, et al. Malignant transformation in synovial chondromatosis of the knee? Knee 2001;8(3):239–42.

28. Kaiser TE, Ivins JC, Unni KK. Malignant transformation of extra-articular synovial chondromatosis: report of a case. Skeletal Radiol 1980;5(4):223–6.

29. Sah AP, Geller DS, Mankin HJ, et al. Malignant transformation of synovial chondromatosis of the shoulder to chondrosarcoma. J Bone Joint Surg Am 2007; 89(6):1321–8.

30. Hamilton A, Davis RI, Nixon JR. Synovial chondrosarcoma complicating synovial chondromatosis. Report of a case and review of the literature. J Bone Joint Surg Am 1987;69(7):1084–8.

31. Campanacci DA, Matera D, Franchi A, et al. Synovial chondrosarcoma of the hip: report of two cases and literature review. Chir Organi Mov 2008;92(3): 139–44.

32. King JW, Spjut HJ, Fechner RE, et al. Synovial chondrosarcoma of the knee joint. J Bone Joint Surg Am 1967;49(7):1309–13.

33. Taconis WK, van der Heul RO, Taminiau AM. Synovial chondrosarcoma: report of a case and review of the literature. Skeletal Radiol 1997;26(11): 682–5.

34. Bertoni F, Unni K, Beabout J, et al. Chondrosarcomas of the synovium. Cancer Chemother Pharmacol 1991;67(1):155–62.

35. Imakiire N, Fujino T, Morii T, et al. Malignant pigmented villonodular synovitis in the knee - report of a case with rapid clinical progression. Open Orthop J 2011; 5:13–6.

36. Yoon HJ, Cho YA, Lee JI, et al. Malignant pigmented villonodular synovitis of the temporomandibular joint with lung metastasis: a case report and review of the literature. Oral Surg Oral Med Oral Pathol Oral Radiol Endod 2011;111(5): e30–6.

37. Bertoni F, Unni KK, Beabout JW, et al. Malignant giant cell tumor of the tendon sheaths and joints (malignant pigmented villonodular synovitis). Am J Surg Pathol 1997;21(2):153–63.

38. Sharma H, Jane MJ, Reid R. Pigmented villonodular synovitis of the foot and ankle: forty years of experience from the Scottish Bone Tumor Registry. J Foot Ankle Surg 2006;45(5):329–36.

39. Buck P, Mickelson MR, Bonfiglio M. Synovial sarcoma: a review of 33 cases. Clin Orthop Relat Res 1981;156:211–5.

40. Krall RA, Kostianovsky M, Patchefsky AS. Synovial sarcoma. A clinical, patho-logical, and ultrastructural study of 26 cases supporting the recognition of a monophasic variant. Am J Surg Pathol 1981;5(2):137–51.

41. Elias D, White L, Simpson D, et al. Osseus invasion by soft-tissue sarcoma: assessment with MR imaging. Radiology 2003;229:145–52.

42. Griffin CA, Emanuel BS. Translocation (X;18) in a synovial sarcoma. Cancer Genet Cytogenet 1987;26(1):181–3.

43. Amary MF, Berisha F, Bernardi FD, et al. Detection of SS18-SSX fusion tran-scripts in formalin-fixed paraffin-embedded neoplasms: analysis of conventional RT-PCR, qRT-PCR and dual color FISH as diagnostic tools for synovial sarcoma. Mod Pathol 2007;20(4):482–96.

44. Cribb GL, Loo SC, Dickinson I. Limb salvage for soft-tissue sarcomas of the foot and ankle. J Bone Joint Surg Br 2010;92(3):424–9.

45. Park SJ, Glinert KD, Staddon AP. Retrospective analysis of 24 synovial cell sarcoma patients treated with doxorubicin and ifosfamide. J Clin Oncol 2010; 28(Suppl): abstract e20508.

46. Krieg AH, Hefti F, Speth BM, et al. Synovial sarcomas usually metastasize after >5 years: a multicenter retrospective analysis with minimum follow-up of 10 years for survivors. Ann Oncol 2011;22(2):458–67.

47. Ptaszyński K, Szumera-Ciećkiewicz A, Zakrzewska K, et al. Her2, EGFR gene amplification and protein expression in synovial sarcoma before and after combined treatment. Pol J Pathol 2009;60(1):10–8.

48. Eggelmeijer F, Macfarlane JD. Polyarthritis as the presenting symptom of the occurrence and recurrence of a laryngeal carcinoma. Ann Rheum Dis 1992; 51(4):556–7.

49. Chakravarty KK, Webley M. Monarthritis: an unusual presentation of renal cell carcinoma. Ann Rheum Dis 1992;51(5):681–2.

50. Newton P, Freemont AT, Noble J, et al. Secondary malignant synovitis: report of three cases and review of the literature. Q J Med 1984;53(209):135–43.

51. Capovilla M, Durlach A, Fourati E, et al. Chronic monoarthritis and previous history of cancer: think about synovial metastasis. Clin Rheumatol 2007;26(1): 60–3.

52. Zissiadis Y. Acute arthritis as an unusual complication of malignancy. Australas Radiol 2000;44(4):474–7.

53. Evans T, Nercessian BM, Sanders KM. Leukemic arthritis. Semin Arthritis Rheum 1994;24(1):48–56.

54. Acree SC, Pullarkat ST, Quismorio FP Jr, et al. Adult leukemic synovitis is asso-ciated with leukemia of monocytic differentiation. J Clin Rheumatol 2011;17(3): 130–4.

55. Krüger R, Oden J, de Leon F, et al. Malignant non-Hodgkin's lymphoma of the joint. Report of two cases, review of the literature and problems of classification. Unfallchirurg 1993;96(10):556–62 [in German].
56. DeVita VT, Lawrence TS, Rosenberg SA. 8th edition. Cancer: principles & practice of oncology, vol. 2. Philadelphia (PA): Wolters Kluwer/Lippincott Williams & Wilkins; 2008.
57. Schoenfeld Y, Gershwin ME. Cancer and autoimmunity. Amsterdam: Elsevier Science B.V; 2000.
58. Zupancic M, Annamalai A, Brenneman J, et al. Migratory polyarthritis as a paraneoplastic syndrome. J Gen Intern Med 2008;23(12):2136–9.
59. Mok C, Kwan Y. Rheumatoid-like polyarthritis as presenting feature of metastatic carcinoma: a case presentation and review of the literature. Clin Rheumatol 2003;22:353–4.
60. Stummvoll G, Aringer M, Machold K, et al. Cancer polyarthritis resembling rheumatoid arthritis as a first sign of hidden neoplasms. Report of two cases and review of the literature. Scand J Rheumatol 2001;30(1):40–4.
61. Baka Z, Barta P, Losonczy G, et al. Specific expression of PAD4 and citrullinated proteins in lung cancer is not associated with anti-CCP antibody production. Int Immunol 2011;23(6):405–14.
62. Glasnovic M, Bedekovic D, Bonsjak I, et al. Arthritis in paraneoplastic syndrome–a way to early cancer diagnosis? A case report. Reumatizam 2009; 56(1):36–40.
63. Brickmann K, Brezinschek R, Yazdani-Biuki B, et al. Superior specificity of anticitrullinated peptide antibodies in patients with chronic lymphocytic leukemia and arthritis. Clin Exp Rheumatol 2010;28(6):888–91.
64. Bizzaro N, Mazzanti G, Tonutti E, et al. Diagnostic accuracy of the anti-citrulline antibody assay for rheumatoid arthritis. Clin Chem 2001;47(6):1089–93.
65. Chakravarty E, Genovese M. Associations between rheumatoid arthritis and malignancy. Rheum Dis Clin North Am 2004;30(2):271–84.
66. Olivieri I, Salvarani C, Cantini F. RS3PE syndrome: an overview. Clin Exp Rheumatol 2000;18(4 Suppl 20):S53–5.
67. Paira S, Graf C, Roverano S, et al. Remitting seronegative symmetrical synovitis with pitting oedema: a study of 12 cases. Clin Rheumatol 2002;21(2): 146–9.
68. Russell EB. Remitting seronegative symmetrical synovitis with pitting edema syndrome: followup for neoplasia. J Rheumatol 2005;32(9):1760–1.
69. Tunc SE, Arslan C, Ayvacioglu NB, et al. Paraneoplastic remitting seronegative symmetrical synovitis with pitting edema (RS3PE syndrome): a report of two cases and review of the literature. Rheumatol Int 2004;24(4):234–7.
70. Hagha H, Eide G, Brun J, et al. Cancer in association with polymyalgia rheumatica and temporal arteritis. J Rheumatol 1993;20:1335–9.
71. Naschitz J, Slobodin G, Yeshurun D, et al. Atypical polymyalgia rheumatica as a presentation of metastatic cancer. Arch Intern Med 1997;157:2381.
72. Naschitz JE. Rheumatic syndromes: clues to occult neoplasia. Curr Opin Rheumatol 2001;13:62–6.
73. Espinosa GFJ, Munoz-Rodriguez FJ, Cervera R, et al. Myelodysplastic and myeloproliferative syndromes associated with giant cell arteritis and polymyalgia rheumatica: a coincidental coexistence or a causal relationship? Clin Rheumatol 2002;21:309–13.
74. Wallach HW. Lupus-like syndrome associated with carcinoma of the breast. Arch Intern Med 1977;137(4):532–5.

75. Hong YH, Lee CK. Autoimmune lymphoproliferative syndrome-like syndrome presented as lupus-like syndrome with mycobacterial joint infection evolved into the lymphoma. Rheumatol Int 2009;29(5):569–73.

76. Hammoudeh M. Acute lymphocytic leukemia presenting as lupus-like syndrome. Rheumatol Int 2006;26:581–2.

77. Hernández Hernández JL, Gutiérrez Polo RA, Sampedro Alvarez JR, et al. A "lupus-like" syndrome as the form of presentation of pulmonary adenocarcinoma. An Med Interna 2000;17(10):558–9.

78. Chtourou M, Aubin F, Savariault I, et al. Digital necrosis and lupus-like syndrome preceding ovarian carcinoma. Dermatology 1998;196(3):348–9.

79. Strickland RW, Limmani A, Wall JG, et al. Hairy cell leukemia presenting as a lupus-like illness. Arthritis Rheum 1988;31(4):566–8.

80. Rogues AM, Vidal E, Boudinet F, et al. Breast cancer with systemic manifestations mimicking Still's disease. J Rheumatol 1993;20(10):1786–7.

81. Ahn J, Oh J, Lee J, et al. Adult onset Still's disease diagnosed concomitantly with occult papillary thyroid cancer: paraneoplastic manifestation or coincidence? Clin Rheumatol 2010;29(2):221–4.

82. Shibuya Y, Matuo K, Kawada T, et al. Adult onset Still's disease associated esophageal cancer: a case report. Ryumachi 2003;43(3):577–82.

83. Kent P, Michet CJ, Luthra H. Relapsing polychondritis. Curr Opin Rheumatol 2004;16:56–61.

84. Bochtler T, Hensel M, Lorenz HM, et al. Chronic lymphocytic leukaemia and concomitant relapsing polychondritis: a report on one treatment for the combined manifestation of two diseases. Rheumatology (Oxford) 2005;44(9):1199.

85. Manghani M, Andrews J, Higgens C. Kaposi's sarcoma in a patient with severe relapsing polychondritis. Rheumatol Int 2004;24(5):309–11.

86. Yanagi T, Matsumura T, Kamekura R, et al. Relapsing polychondritis and malignant lymphoma: is polychondritis paraneoplastic? Arch Dermatol 2007;143(1):89–90.

87. Labarthe MP, Bayle-Lebey P, Bazex J. Cutaneous manifestations of relapsing polychondritis in a patient receiving goserelin for carcinoma of the prostate. Dermatology 1997;195(4):391–4.

88. Johnson JJ, Leonard-Segal A, Nashel DJ. Jaccoud's-type arthropathy: an association with malignancy. J Rheumatol 1989;16(9):1278–80.

89. Hickling P, Wilkins M, Newman GR, et al. A study of amyloid arthropathy in multiple myeloma. Q J Med 1981;50:417–33.

90. Cohen AS, Canoso JJ. Rheumatological aspects of amyloid disease. Clin Rheum Dis 1975;1:149–61.

91. Terkeltaub R. Clinical practice. Gout. N Engl J Med 2003;349(17):1647–55.

92. Pavithran K, Thomas M. Chronic myeloid leukemia presenting as gout. Clin Rheumatol 2001;20(4):288–9.

93. Yu T, Weinreb N, Wittman R, et al. Secondary gout associated with chronic myeloproliferative disorders. Semin Arthritis Rheum 1976;5(3):247–56.

94. Tsimberidou AM, Keating MJ. Hyperuricemic syndromes in cancer patients. Contrib Nephrol 2005;147:47–60.

95. Zhang W, Doherty M, Bardin T, et al. European League Against Rheumatism recommendations for calcium pyrophosphate deposition. Part I: terminology and diagnosis. Ann Rheum Dis 2011;70(4):563–70.

96. Clines GA, Guise TA. Hypercalcemia of malignancy. In: Medical care of cancer patients. Shelton (CT): BC Decker Inc; 2009. p. 188–193.

97. Rosenthal A. Pathogenesis of calcium pyrophosphate crystal deposition disease. Curr Rheumatol Rep 2011;3(1):17–23.

98. Zhang W, Doherty M, Pascual E, et al. EULAR recommendations for calcium pyrophosphate deposition. Part II: management. Ann Rheum Dis 2011;70(4): 571–5.

99. Martinez-Lavin M, Pineda C, Valdez T, et al. Primary hypertrophic osteoarthropathy. Semin Arthritis Rheum 1988;17:156–62.

100. Naschitz J, Rosner I, Rozenbaum M, et al. Cancer-associated rheumatic disorders: clues to occult neoplasia. Semin Arthritis Rheum 1995;24:231–41.

101. Donnelly B, Johnson P. Detection of hypertrophic pulmonary osteoarthropathy of skeletal imaging with 99mTc-labeled diphosphonate. Radiology 1975;114: 389–91.

102. Segal A, Mackenzie A. Hypertrophic osteoarthropathy: a 10-year retrospective analysis. Semin Arthritis Rheum 1982;12:220–32.

103. Yao Q, Altman RD, Brahn E. Periostitis and hypertrophic pulmonary osteoarthropathy: report of 2 cases and review of the literature. Semin Arthritis Rheum 2009;38:458–66.

104. Shih W. Pulmonary hypertrophic osteoarthropathy and its resolution. Semin Nucl Med 2004;34:159–63.

105. Yeo W, Leung SF, Chan AT, et al. Radiotherapy for extreme hypertrophic pulmonary osteoarthropathy associated with malignancy. Clin Oncol (R Coll Radiol) 1996;8:195–7.

106. Morita M, Sakaguchi Y, Kuma S, et al. Hypertrophic osteoarthropathy associated with esophageal cancer. Ann Thorac Surg 2003;76:1744–6.

107. Alonso-Bartolomé P, Martínez-Taboada V, Pina T, et al. Hypertrophic osteoarthropathy secondary to vascular prosthesis infection: report of 3 cases and review of the literature. Medicine (Baltimore) 2006;85: 183–91.

108. Treasure T. Hypertrophic pulmonary osteoarthropathy and the vagus nerve: an historical note. J R Soc Med 2006;99:388–90.

109. Silveri F, De Angelis R, Argentati F, et al. Hypertrophic osteoarthropathy: endothelium and platelet function. Clin Rheumatol 1996;15(5):435–9.

110. Nguyen S, Hojjati M. Review of current therapies for secondary hypertrophic pulmonary osteoarthropathy. Clin Rheumatol 2011;30:7–13.

111. Guyot-Drouot M, Solau-Gervais E, Cortet B, et al. Rheumatologic manifestations of pachydermoperiostosis and preliminary experience with bisphosphonates. J Rheumatol 2000;27:2418–23.

112. Slobodin G, Rosner I, Feld J, et al. Pamidronate treatment in rheumatology practice: a comprehensive review. Clin Rheumatol 2009;28:1359.

113. King M, Nelson D. Hypertrophic osteoarthropathy effectively treated with zoledronic acid. Clin Lung Cancer 2008;9:179.

114. Carsons S. The association of malignancy with rheumatic and connective tissue diseases. Semin Oncol 1997;24(3):360.

115. Shiel WJ, Prete P, Jason M, et al. Palmar fasciitis and arthritis with ovarian and non-ovarian carcinoma: New syndrome. Am J Med 1985;79:640–4.

116. Willemse P, Mulder N, van der Tempel H, et al. Palmar fascitis and arthritis in a patient with extra-ovarian adenocarcinoma of the coelomic epithelium. Ann Rheum Dis 1991;50:53–4.

117. Enomoto M, Takemura H, Suzuki M, et al. Palmar fasciitis and polyarthritis associated with gastric carcinoma: complete resolution after total gastrectomy. Intern Med 2000;39:754.

118. Alexandroff A, Hazleman B, Matthewson M, et al. Woody hands. Lancet 2003; 361:1344.
119. Tannenbaum H, Anderson LG, Schur PH. Association of polyarthritis, subcutaneous nodules, and pancreatic disease. J Rheumatol 1975;2(1):15–20.
120. Virshup A, Sliwinski A. Polyarthritis and subcutaneous nodules associated with carcinoma of the pancreas. Arthritis Rheum 1973;16:388–92.
121. Dahl PR, Su WP, Cullimore KC, et al. Pancreatic panniculitis. J Am Acad Dermatol 1995;33(3):413.
122. García-Romero D, Vanaclocha F. Pancreatic panniculitis. Dermatol Clin 2008; 26(4):465.
123. Luz F, Gaspar T, Kalil-Gaspar N, et al. Multicentric reticulohistiocytosis. J Eur Acad Dermatol Venereol 2001;15(6):524–31.
124. Barrow M, Holubar K. Multicentric reticulohistiocytosis. A review of 33 patients. Medicine (Baltimore) 1969;48(4):287–305.
125. Ginsburg W, O'Duffy J, Morris J, et al. Multicentric reticulohistiocytosis: response to alkylating agents in six patients. Ann Intern Med 1989;11(5):384–8.
126. Gourmelen O, Le Loët X, Fortier-Beaulieu M, et al. Methotrexate treatment of multicentric reticulohistiocytosis. J Rheumatol 1991;18(4):627–8.
127. Matejicka CG, Morgan J, Schlegelmilch JG. Multicentric reticulohistiocytosis treated successfully with an anti-tumor necrosis factor agent: comment on the article by Gorman et al. Arthritis Rheum 2003;48:864–6.
128. Kovach B, Calamia K, Walsh J, et al. Treatment of multicentric reticulohistiocytosis with etanercept. Arch Dermatol 2004;140(8):919–21.
129. Kaandorp CJ, Krijnen P, Moens HJ, et al. The outcome of bacterial arthritis: a prospective community-based study. Arthritis Rheum 1997;40(5):884–92.
130. Goldenberg DL. Septic arthritis. Lancet 1998;351:197–202.
131. Fallon SM, Guzik HJ, Kramer LE. *Clostridium septicum* arthritis associated with colonic carcinoma. J Rheumatol 1986;13(3):662–3.
132. Lyon LJ, Nevins MA. Carcinoma of the colon presenting as pyogenic arthritis. JAMA 1979;241(19):2060.
133. Dylewski J, Luterman L. Septic arthritis and *Clostridium septicum*: a clue to colon cancer. CMAJ 2010;182(13):1446–7.
134. Cuéllar ML, Silveira LH, Espinoza LR. Fungal arthritis. Ann Rheum Dis 1992; 51(5):690–7.
135. Meier JF, Beekmann SE. Mycobacterial and fungal infections of bone and joints. Curr Opin Rheumatol 1995;7:329–36.
136. Pfaller MA, Pappas PG, Wingard JR. Invasive fungal pathogens: current epidemiological trends. Clin Infect Dis 2006;43:S3–14.
137. Hu XR, He JS, Ye XJ, et al. *Candida tropicalis* arthritis in a patient with acute leukemia. Zhongguo Shi Yan Xue Ye Xue Za Zhi 2008;16(5):1215–8.
138. Nguyen VQ, Penn RL. *Candida krusei* infectious arthritis. A rare complication of neutropenia. Am J Med 1987;83(5):963–5.
139. Pemán J, Jarque I, Bosch M, et al. Spondylodiscitis caused by *Candida krusei*: case report and susceptibility patterns. J Clin Microbiol 2006;44(5): 1912–4.
140. Sili U, Yilmaz M, Ferhanoglu B, et al. *Candida krusei* arthritis in a patient with hematologic malignancy: successful treatment with voriconazole. Clin Infect Dis 2007;45(7):897–8.
141. Vicari P, Feitosa Pinheiro R, Chauffaille Mde L, et al. Septic arthritis as the first sign of *Candida tropicalis* fungaemia in an acute lymphoid leukemia patient. Braz J Infect Dis 2003;7(6):426–8.

142. Wang HP, Yen YF, Chen WS, et al. An unusual case of *Candida tropicalis* and *Candida krusei* arthritis in a patient with acute myelogenous leukemia before chemotherapy. Clin Rheumatol 2007;26(7):1195–7.
143. Ioannou Y, Isenberg DA. Current evidence for the induction of autoimmune rheumatic manifestations by cytokine therapy. Arthritis Rheum 2000;43(7): 1431–42.
144. Hory B, Blanc D, Saint-Hilier Y. Systemic lupus erythematosus-like syndrome induced by alpha-interferon therapy. Eur J Med 1992;1(6):379.
145. Koch B, Kranzhöfer N, Pfreundschu M, et al. First manifestations of seronegative spondylarthropathy following autologous stem cell transplantation in HLA-B27-positive patients. Bone Marrow Transplant 2000;26(6):673–5.
146. Onur O, Celiker R. Polyarthritis as a complication of intravesical bacillus Calmette-Guerin immunotherapy for bladder cancer. Clin Rheumatol 1999; 18(1):74–6.
147. Crew KD, Greenlee H, Capodice J, et al. Prevalence of joint symptoms in post-menopausal women taking aromatase inhibitors for early-stage breast cancer. J Clin Oncol 2007;25(25):3877–83.
148. Warner E, Keshavjee al-N, Shupak R, et al. Rheumatic symptoms following adjuvant therapy for breast cancer. Am J Clin Oncol 1997;20(3):322–6.
149. Loprinzi CL, Maddocks-Christianson K, Wolf SL, et al. The Paclitaxel acute pain syndrome: sensitization of nociceptors as the putative mechanism. Cancer J 2007;13(6):399–403.

Neoplastic/ Paraneoplastic Dermatitis, Fasciitis, and Panniculitis

Anjali Shah, MD[a], Alexander Jack, MD[b], Helen Liu, MD[b],
R. Samuel Hopkins, MD[b],*

KEYWORDS

- Skin • Paraneoplastic • Dermatoses • Malignancy
- Dermatology

Changes of the epidermis, dermis, and subcutaneous fat can occur in the setting of internal malignancy. When a particular cutaneous disorder is strongly associated with, and parallels the course of, the internal malignancy, it is considered a paraneoplastic dermatosis. Recognizing such cutaneous clues may lead to early identification of the underlying malignancy, because the skin findings often precede the diagnosis of malignancy. This article discusses several characteristic skin presentations associated with internal malignancy. These disorders are organized into superficial (changes of the epidermis and dermis) and deep (changes of the fat and fascia) dermatoses.

EPIDERMAL AND DERMAL MANIFESTATIONS OF INTERNAL MALIGNANCY
Tripe Palms

Tripe palms (TP), initially described by Clarke[1] in 1977, is a rare paraneoplastic dermatosis with roughly 100 cases described in the literature.[2,3] Clinically, patients present with hyperkeratosis and accentuation of skin ridges on the palms and, at times, the soles. The skin has a rugose, velvety appearance, said to resemble tripe, a food prepared from bovine foregut (**Fig. 1A**). Changes are exaggerated over pressure points, such as the fingertips and thenar and hypothenar eminences. Diffuse involvement of the palms with either a mosslike or honeycomb pattern has been described.[1,4]

The authors have nothing to disclose, and there was no funding support for this paper.
[a] Division of Dermatology, Department of Medicine, Loyola University Medical Center, Room 101, Building 54, 2160 South First Avenue, Maywood, IL 60153, USA
[b] Department of Dermatology, Oregon Health & Science University, 3303 Southwest Bond Avenue, Mail Code 16D, Portland, OR 97239, USA
* Corresponding author.
E-mail address: hopkirob@ohsu.edu

Rheum Dis Clin N Am 37 (2011) 573–592
doi:10.1016/j.rdc.2011.09.003
0889-857X/11/$ – see front matter © 2011 Elsevier Inc. All rights reserved.

rheumatic.theclinics.com

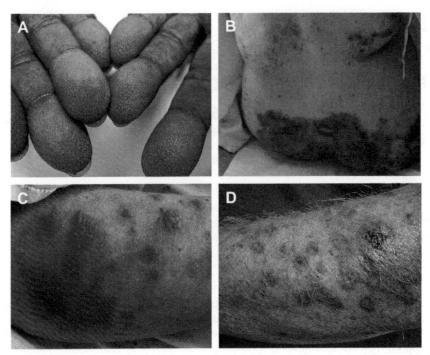

Fig. 1. (*A*) TP; (*B*) necrolytic migratory erythema; (*C*) Sweet's syndrome (*D*) necrobiotic xanthogranuloma.

Associated pruritus occurs in 25%.[5] When clubbing of the nails is seen with TP (18% of cases), a pulmonary carcinoma should be suspected as the underlying malignancy.[6]

TP is more common in men than women, and is found almost exclusively in adults. There is no known genetic association or racial predilection.[7] Whether TP is a distinct entity or a manifestation of malignant acanthosis nigricans on the palms is contested; some investigators contend that TP, malignant acanthosis nigricans, and the sign of Leser-Trélat (LT) are not separate entities but rather exist on a spectrum.[2,8] Most cases of TP are associated with malignancy (94% of cases) and malignant acanthosis nigricans frequently coexists (77% of cases).[2] TP frequently develops before the diagnosis of malignancy, but may occur concurrently or after the diagnosis of cancer. When present alone, TP is most commonly associated with pulmonary carcinoma, followed in incidence by gastric carcinoma. However, when present with acanthosis nigricans, a gastric carcinoma is more common. Tumors of the genitourinary tract, tongue, and breast have also been associated with TP.[7]

Treatment is difficult and is primarily aimed at the underlying tumor. In one-third of cases, TP parallels the course of the associated malignancy.[9] Retinoids, emollients, keratolytics, and topical steroids, although reported, are often of limited benefit.[10,11]

Acanthosis Nigricans

Although benign acanthosis nigricans (typically familial or associated with obesity or endocrinopathy) is common, malignant acanthosis nigricans (MAN) is rare, with roughly 1000 cases reported in the literature.[12] MAN usually occurs in adults more than 40 years of age.[13] There is no known genetic, racial, or gender predilection.[7,14]

Clinically, MAN usually presents with a sudden onset of symmetric, hyperpigmented, thickened plaques creating a velvety texture. Plaques may be yellow, gray, or black.[15] MAN most commonly affects the nape and sides of the neck, the axillae, inframammary folds, and inguinal creases. Frequently, acrochordons (skin tags) are seen within the plaques.[8] MAN has been associated with florid cutaneous papillomatosis[16] and often occurs in conjunction with TP and/or the sign of LT.[5]

In contrast with benign acanthosis nigricans, MAN is usually extensive and rapidly progressive. Forty-one percent have associated generalized pruritus.[14] With extensive involvement, lesions may involve the areola and umbilicus. Mucosal involvement occurs in 35% of patients with MAN, and may affect the eyes, oral cavity (including lips, gingival, buccal mucosa and palate), esophagus, larynx, and anal and genital mucosa.[7]

MAN may either precede (18%), accompany (61%), or follow (21%) the onset of the internal cancer.[17] Most cases are associated with adenocarcinoma, especially of the gastrointestinal tract (60% stomach), lung, and breast. Cancers of the gallbladder, pancreas, esophagus, liver, prostate, kidney, colon, rectum, uterus, and ovaries have also been reported,[7] as well as hepatocellular cancer[18] and lymphoma.[19]

MAN tends to parallel the course of the associated malignancy. Skin changes usually regress with suppression or removal of underlying malignancy, and, conversely, worsen following relapse.[15] The overall prognosis for most patients with MAN is poor because the associated tumors are usually aggressive with a high mortality.[14]

The Sign of LT

The sign of LT is a rapid appearance or growth of multiple seborrheic keratoses associated with an underlying malignancy.[20] It is named after the surgeons Leser and Trélat who first independently described the occurrence of skin lesions with an internal malignancy in 1890.[21] However, it is now thought that the lesions they were describing were vascular angiomas, and it was Hollander[22] who first associated seborrheic keratoses with malignancy in 1900. Controversy exists regarding the validity of this sign because both seborrheic keratoses and internal malignancy are common in the elderly population, making it difficult to distinguish coincidence from correlation. In addition, determining whether seborrheic keratoses are eruptive can be difficult, because an exact definition is lacking.[23]

Clinically, LT presents as multiple, eruptive seborrheic keratoses primarily on the trunk and extremities. Individual lesions are clinically and pathologically indistinguishable from the common seborrheic keratosis. Pruritus is found 26% to 51% of the time.[24,25]

The sign of LT is rare, with roughly 100 cases reported to date. The average age of onset is 60 years, although young patients have been reported.[26] There is no gender or racial predilection. Sixty-five percent of patients with LT have a concurrent paraneoplastic dermatosis, with MAN occurring 29% of the time.[23]

Similar to MAN, the most common type of underlying tumors are adenocarcinomas, especially of the gastrointestinal tract (32%). Unlike MAN, lymphoproliferative disorders are the next most commonly associated malignancy, occurring 21% of the time.[25] Both MAN and LT have been associated with aggressive malignancies. Metastases were found 57% of the time when the sign of LT was present.[23]

Although treatment is directed at the underlying malignancy, in 60% of cases of LT, the cutaneous findings do not parallel the course of the cancer.[23] Local treatment of the seborrheic keratoses, such as shave removal or cryotherapy, can be performed for irritating lesions.[25]

Bazex Syndrome (Acrokeratosis Paraneoplastica)

Acrokeratosis paraneoplastica, or Bazex syndrome, is a paraneoplastic process that was named after Bazex in 1965, who described a patient with scaly erythematous lesions of the extremities who had an underlying squamous cell carcinoma of the piriform fossa.[27] Clinically, the lesions present as symmetric psoriasiform plaques, most commonly on the nose, helices, earlobes, and distal extremities. Nail dystrophy is often present, and, in advanced disease, the skin lesions can spread to involve the elbows, knees, thighs, and arms. Palmar and plantar keratoderma, accentuated in areas of pressure, may also be seen.[28] Bullous, vesicular, and pustular lesions have been reported.[29,30]

Bazex syndrome almost always occurs in men older than 40 years, and predominantly in white men.[27,28] HLA typing in several cases has shown HLA-A2 and or B8 to be present.[31,32] A history of smoking or alcohol use is common. The rash often mimics seborrheic dermatitis, lupus erythematosus, or psoriasis, which may lead to underdiagnosis of this syndrome.

Bazex syndrome is always associated with an underlying malignancy. The cutaneous findings most commonly precede the diagnosis of malignancy (two-thirds of the time); however, the eruption may occur simultaneously or after the malignancy is discovered.[28]

The most common types of malignancies associated with Bazex are squamous cell carcinomas (64% of cases) from the upper aerodigestive tract, most commonly from the oral cavity, larynx, pharynx, lung, and esophagus. Lymph node metastases are present in 50% of cases, with some cases presenting with cervical lymph node metastases of unknown primary (16%).[32] Concurrent acquired ichthyosis (AI) and the sign of LT have been reported.[33]

In more than 90% of cases, the cutaneous findings parallel the course of the cancer.[28] Removal of the tumor usually causes regression, and worsening may herald a recurrence. Treatment with keratolytics, topical steroids, and antibiotics does not show improvement in most cases.[32] There have been some reports of improvement with psoralen and ultraviolet A therapy[29] and oral retinoids,[34] but treating the underlying malignancy is the primary management.

Acquired Ichthyosis

Ichthyosis is derived from the Greek word for fish, *ichthys*, and describes the resemblance of the skin in this disease to fish scales.[35] Ichthyosis can be genetic or acquired, and the acquired forms are secondary to a variety of different drugs and diseases, including malignancy.[36] In 1943, Ronchese[37] first described a patient with Hodgkin disease who later developed AI. Subsequent case reports have described AI as a paraneoplastic dermatosis.

AI most commonly manifests in adulthood and is otherwise difficult to distinguish from the hereditary forms of ichthyosis.[38] Symmetric scaling is seen, which ranges in severity from minor roughness and dryness to severe desquamation and platelike scaling. The color of the scales varies from white to gray to brown, with a diameter ranging from less than 1 mm to greater than 1 cm. It primarily affects the trunk and limbs, typically being accentuated on the extensor surfaces with relative sparing of the flexures. AI usually affects the lower extremities more significantly than the upper extremities.[39] AI may be more common in men than women.[40] There is no reported genetic or racial predilection.[7]

AI usually presents after the diagnosis of the malignancy, but it may present before.[35] The most common associated malignancy is Hodgkin disease, estimated to occur in 60% to 80% of cases.[7,41,42] Other lymphoproliferative malignancies and solid organ tumors have been reported. AI has been seen in conjunction with other paraneoplastic dermatoses such as Bazex syndrome,[43] erythema gyratum repens,[44] and dermatomyositis.[45]

As with the other paraneoplastic dermatoses, management of AI is designed to treat the underlying tumor. The course of the disease usually parallels the underlying malignancy, and most cases of tumor remission result in resolution of the ichthyosis.[35,46] Topical steroids, keratolytics, and oral retinoids have been tried with variable success.[47,48]

Erythema Gyratum Repens

Erythema gyratum repens (EGR) is derived from the Greek word *gyrate*, meaning circle, and the Latin word *repens*, meaning to creep. The first case was reported in 1952 when Gammel[49] described a "knotty cypress wood grain" pruritic eruption associated with adenocarcinoma of the breast that resolved following tumor removal.

Clinically, the eruption involves concentric erythematous rings that develop trailing scale at their edges and advance at a rapid rate ($\sim$1 cm per day). The classic woodgrain scaling is often associated with pruritus, ichthyosis, and palmoplantar keratoderma. At times, a peripheral eosinophilia is seen.[50] Men are affected twice as commonly as women, with an average age of 63 years at onset. All cases but 1[51] have been described in white people.[50,52]

EGR is associated with an internal malignancy more than 80% of the time. EGR usually precedes the diagnosis of malignancy by an average of 9 months. Rarely, the skin eruption follows the diagnosis of malignancy.[50,53] Approximately 33% of patients have an underlying lung cancer, 8% esophageal cancer, 6% breast cancer, and another 6% with an unknown primary.[49,52] Other solid organ and lymphoproliferative malignancies have been reported.[54]

Although therapies directed at the skin changes are typically ineffective, EGR characteristically improves with successful treatment of the underlying malignancy. Systemic steroids have shown variable success.[55] EGR may resolve immediately before death, possibly because of generalized antemortem immunosuppression.[52]

Necrolytic Migratory Erythema (Glucagonoma Syndrome)

Necrolytic migratory erythema (NME) is a rare cutaneous dermatitis that is most often seen with glucagonoma syndrome. Glucagonoma syndrome is a paraneoplastic syndrome with a characteristic triad of a pancreatic tumor secreting glucagon, hyperglycemia, and NME. In 1942, Becker and colleagues[56] first described the association of an erosive erythema occurring with a pancreatic neoplasm. In 1966, McGavran and colleagues[57] attributed the syndrome to hyperglucagonemia, and, in 1973, the term NME was coined by Wilkinson[58,59] to describe the characteristic associated cutaneous eruption. In a review of 21 patients with glucagonoma syndrome, all of the patients had NME at one point in their illness, and 67% had NME as the presenting complaint.[60]

Clinically, patients often present emaciated, with a chronic dermatitis of many years. In many instances, they have been misdiagnosed with eczema, acrodermatitis enteropathica, or seborrheic dermatitis on presentation. The skin eruption is characterized by a pattern of spontaneous remissions and exacerbations without identifiable triggering factors. It can be highly pruritic and painful, and most commonly involves the intertriginous areas, perineum, lower extremities, and buttocks. The lesions often begin as erythematous macules, papules, and patches that evolve into annular or circinate well-demarcated plaques. There can be fragile vesicles and bullae in the central portion of the lesions, which leave extensive painful erosions when damaged. Other mucocutaneous manifestations may include angular stomatitis, cheilosis, painful glossitis, blepharitis, conjunctivitis, perianal and genital lesions, alopecia, and nail dystrophy (see **Fig. 1**B).[60–63]

Associated clinical features of the glucagonoma syndrome include weight loss (71%), normocytic anemia (43%–90%), diarrhea (15%–29%), neurologic and psychiatric symptom and signs (20%), and thromboembolic phenomena (11%–14%).[60,63–65] Less than 250 cases of NME have been reported in the literature since 1942. The prevalence is equal in men and women, and most commonly presents in the sixth decade of life.[66]

NME is unique among paraneoplastic syndromes, because it is specific for a particular tumor (glucagonoma) when found in the glucagonoma syndrome. Glucagonoma, an α-cell tumor of the pancreas, is most often identified in the body and tail of the pancreas.[64] At least 50% of tumors are metastatic at the time of diagnosis. The most common site for metastasis is the liver, followed by regional lymph nodes, bone, adrenal gland, kidney, and lung.[63,67] In a recent series, the 10-year survival rate in 233 patients with glucagonomas was 51.6% in those with metastases and 64.3% in those without metastases.[68]

NME has also been reported in the absence of the pancreatic tumor, which has been termed pseudoglucagonoma syndrome. Pseudoglucagonoma is typically seen in association with intestinal malabsorption disorders, cirrhosis, inflammatory bowel disease, and pancreatitis.[69]

Surgical removal of the tumor is the most effective treatment, which may produce rapid clinical resolution of the rash.[63,70] Supplementation with zinc, amino acids, and essential fatty acids, and long-acting somatostatin analogues such as octreotide, may also be beneficial.[71,72]

Dermatomyositis

Dermatomyositis (DM) is an idiopathic inflammatory myopathy often causing patients to present with characteristic cutaneous findings and proximal muscle weakness. The association of dermatomyositis with malignancy was first reported by Stertz in 1916,[73] who described a patient with proximal muscle weakness, eyelid changes, and evidence of myositis on muscle biopsy, as well as a coexisting gastric carcinoma.[73]

Gottron papules and a heliotrope rash are pathognomonic of dermatomyositis. Other findings may include periungual telangiectasia;, cuticular overgrowth; nailfold infarcts; poikiloderma, especially over the extensor extremities; a scaly scalp dermatitis; and/or photosensitivity accompanied by proximal muscle weakness. Dermatomyositis is a multisystem disorder and can be associated with several systemic manifestations.[52,74,75]

In a review of 42 retrospective case series on inflammatory myopathies, 24% of patients with DM had an associated malignancy.[74] The linkage of HLADqA1*0301 with anti-p155/140 antibodies in white patients with myositis suggests a possible genetic basis.[76]

Although dermatomyositis may occur before, after, or concurrent with the diagnosis of cancer, the risk of malignancy is greatest within the first 3 years of diagnosis of DM.[77,78] The most common malignancies are ovarian, lung, gastrointestinal tract, and breast in Western countries; nasopharyngeal carcinoma is commonly associated in certain Asian and African countries.[74] Other reported malignancies include angiotropic lymphoma, urachal carcinoma, and prostate cancer.[52]

Because the risk of an underlying malignancy is significant in patients with DM, an extensive evaluation for malignancy is advisable. The patient's individual risk factors and the most commonly associated malignancies should guide this evaluation. Factors that predict malignancy include cutaneous necrosis, more severe muscle disease refractory to steroid therapy,[79] and the absence of overlap connective tissue disease features.[74] Anti-p155/140 antibodies have a predictive value for malignancy in adult patients.[80]

Andras and colleagues[81] reported remission of the myositis in 16 of 22 patients after treatment of the underlying malignancy. In addition to treatment of the primary tumor, systemic immunosuppressive agents may improve the associated myopathy; sun protection, topical steroids, and immunosuppressives may benefit the cutaneous manifestations.[81,82]

Paraneoplastic Pemphigus

Classically, pemphigus refers to mucocutaneous diseases that are characterized by intraepithelial blisters, caused by a loss of normal cell-cell adhesion secondary to autoantibodies against cell-surface proteins. The concept of paraneoplastic pemphigus (PNP) was solidified in the early 1990s when it was observed that an underlying neoplasm was always associated with a certain set of clinically atypical pemphigus patients.[83] In two-thirds of patients, the disease presents before the neoplasm is recognized.[84] The mean age of onset is 59 years and there is no gender predominance.[85]

Clinically, PNP is characterized by severe and intractable stomatitis, along with polymorphic cutaneous eruptions ranging from lichen planus–like or erythema multiforme–like lesions, to the more well-recognized bullae of classic pemphigus.[86] Compared with pemphigus vulgaris, PNP is more likely to involve acral skin.[84] In adults, the most commonly associated malignancies are non-Hodgkin lymphoma and chronic lymphocytic leukemia, and, to a lesser extent, Castleman disease, thymomas, sarcomas, and Waldenstrom macroglobulinemia.[84] In children and adolescents, the associated underlying neoplasm is predominantly Castleman disease.[87]

Immunoglobulin G (IgG) autoantibodies against multiple epithelial proteins critical to cell-cell adhesion (including desmosomes and hemidesmosomes) develop in patients with PNP. These autoantibodies include desmoplakins I and II, bullous pemphigoid antigen 1, envoplakin, periplakin, plectin, and desmoglein 1 and 3.[84] Serum autoantibodies against the plakin proteins are the most diagnostic markers.

Prognosis is poor, and the disease is highly resistant to many immunosuppressive therapies. First-line treatment remains oral corticosteroids, and combination therapy with cyclophosphamide, high-dose intravenous immunoglobulin (IVIG) and/or rituximab is often required.[88] However, even if resolution of the mucocutaneous features of PNP is achieved with successful treatment of the underlying malignancy and immunosuppressive therapy, some patients may develop, and ultimately succumb to, progressive constrictive bronchiolitis obliterans, the cause of which is unclear.[89]

Sweet's Syndrome

Sweet's syndrome is the prototype of the neutrophilic dermatoses, and is characterized by the constellation of pyrexia, neutrophilia, tender erythematous cutaneous lesions, and prompt response to corticosteroids. The disease was first described in association with aerodigestive tract infections,[90] and currently is best classified under 3 clinical settings[91]: classic or idiopathic (most frequently associated with streptococcus and yersinia infections, inflammatory bowel disease, or pregnancy), malignancy associated (most commonly acute myelogenous leukemia), and drug induced (most clearly associated with granulocyte-colony stimulating factor and all-transretinoic acid).

Although idiopathic Sweet's affects predominantly young women, malignancy-associated Sweet's affects middle-aged men and women equally, and accounts for about 20% to 30% of cases.[92,93] Besides acute myelogenous leukemia, Sweet's has been reported with lymphomas, chronic leukemias, myelomas, myelodysplastic syndromes, and a variety of solid tumors (eg, breast and colon).[94] In 60% of cases, the onset of Sweet's syndrome either precedes or coincides with the discovery of a neoplasm.[93]

Patients typically present with tender, pseudovesicular, or crusted erythematous plaques on the head, neck, and upper extremities, which tend to resolve without scarring (see **Fig. 1**C).[91] A nonspecific flulike illness often precedes skin lesions and fever typically develops. The plaques occasionally exhibit true vesicles, bullae, or pustules. In the setting of malignancy, more widespread involvement may be seen. Atypical presentations, such as vesiculobullous lesions and oral pustular lesions that may progress to ulceration, may occur in hematologic disorders such as myelodysplastic syndromes and myelogenous leukemia.[92] Pathergy, the onset of lesions at sites of trauma (eg, needle sticks), is common. Extracutaneous involvement may occur, including involvement of the eyes, lungs, bones, heart, muscle, and central nervous system. Constitutionally, patients may appear very ill, and complain of arthralgias, malaise, headache, and myalgias. Although a peripheral neutrophilia is characteristic, its absence does not exclude the diagnosis, because patients with neutropenia associated with their leukemia or its treatment may develop Sweet's.[95]

The treatment of choice is systemic corticosteroids. Potassium iodide and colchicine are alternative first-line therapies. Second-line agents include indomethacin, clofazimine, cyclosporine, and dapsone.[96] Recurrence is common, especially in malignancy-associated Sweet's, and may herald relapse of the underlying cancer.

Necrobiotic Xanthogranuloma

Necrobiotic xanthogranuloma (NXG) is a slowly progressive multiorgan, histiocytic dermatosis associated with paraproteinemia. Clinically, patients present with multiple indurated yellow or violaceous papules and plaques that often involve the periorbital skin. Central atrophy, telangiectasias, ulceration, and scarring may be seen.[97] Lesions may also develop elsewhere on the face, as well as the trunk and proximal extremities (see **Fig. 1**D), and may form within scars. Extracutaneous involvement most commonly involves the eye (in up to 81% of patients)[98]; findings include orbital masses, ectropion, keratitis, and proptosis. Postmortem examination has shown internal organ involvement in NXG, including endocardial lesions. The mean age of onset is 60 years without any gender predilection. Only 75 cases have been reported to date.

A paraproteinemia can be detected in 80% of cases, with IgG-κ monoclonal gammopathy predominating (65%).[98] NXG may be associated with multiple myeloma, plasma cell dyscrasias, and, less frequently, lymphoproliferative disorders and solid tumor malignancies.[99] Roughly one-quarter of patients with associated paraproteinemias go on to develop multiple myeloma.[98,99]

Treatments with reported benefit in NXG include low-dose chlorambucil, melphalan, cyclophosphamide, radiation, and plasmapheresis. Excision carries a high local recurrence rate (42%) and should be avoided.[98] NXG is typically chronic and progressive. Overall survival is good, but prognosis depends on the degree of extracutaneous involvement and the presence and severity of associated malignancies.

Multicentric Reticulohistiocytosis

The term multicentric reticulohistiocytosis (MRH) was first used by Goltz and Laymon[100] in 1954 to describe cases of non–Langerhan cell reticulohistiocytosis with both cutaneous and systemic manifestations. Characteristic skin lesions and a destructive polyarthritis define this condition. Clinically, firm, skin-colored to red-brown papules and nodules develop over acral surfaces (eg, hands, ears), the head, and skin overlying joints. Alignment of small papules periungually can be seen, referred to as the coral bead sign. A symmetric, erosive arthritis of multiple joints develops and may progress to arthritis mutilans.[97] The joints of the fingers, hands, wrists, and knees are preferentially involved. MRH most commonly affects white women in the fourth decade.

Between 15% and 30% of cases are associated with an underlying malignancy, typically solid tumors of the lung, breast, stomach, or cervix, warranting a malignancy work-up in all patients. However, the course of the skin disease does not parallel the course of the underlying neoplasm and thus some have negated the categorization of this disease as paraneoplastic.[101] The mononuclear cells of this disease exhibit properties of osteoclasts such as the tissue lytic markers of tartrate-resistant acid phosphatase and cathepsin K, and RANKL (receptor activator of nuclear factor κ-B ligand).[102] It has been postulated that histiocytes in MRH may differentiate into osteoclastlike multinucleated giant cells in the skin.[103]

Traditionally, methotrexate, either as sole therapy or in combination with other immunosuppressants, has been the mainstay of treatment.[104] Recently, increased levels of tumor necrosis factor (TNF)α and interleukin (IL)-1β within the synovial fluid of patients with MRH have been shown[105] and a few cases of successful treatment with TNFα antagonists have been reported.[106] Case reports and clinical evidence is starting to accumulate on the use of bisphosphonates in this disease, which may act directly on the mononuclear cells leading to inhibition of RANKL, and therefore inhibiting differentiation of histiocytes into osteoclastlike cells.[107,108] Although the disease usually spontaneously remits, the destructive cutaneous and articular lesions may lead to significant disfigurement.

Scleromyxedema

Scleromyxedema, or generalized lichen myxedematosus, is one of the mucinous deposition disorders. Diagnosis of scleromyxedema should fulfill the following criteria: (1) generalized papular and sclerodermoid eruption; (2) skin biopsy showing mucin deposition, fibroblast proliferation, and fibrosis; (3) monoclonal gammopathy (IgG-λ paraproteinemia); and (4) the absence of thyroid disease.[109]

Clinically, numerous waxy, firm, tiny papules develop symmetrically and affected areas of skin become sclerotic. The head and neck, hands, upper trunk, and extremities are typically involved.[110] Longitudinal furrows of the glabella and thickened skin with central depressions over the proximal interphalangeal joints (doughnut sign) are characteristic features. Systemic manifestations in scleromyxedema are prevalent, and can resemble those of scleroderma or other rheumatologic diseases.[111] With disease progression, gradual restriction of movement may occur. In contrast with scleroderma, the skin is moveable over the subcutis, and periungual telangiectasias are absent.[112]

Paraproteinemia, most commonly monoclonal IgG-λ,[109,112] is present in approximately 80% of patients. It does not represent a primary plasma cell dyscrasia, and less than 10% of patients progress to multiple myeloma. There are rare case reports of association with myopathy, including dermatomyositis,[113] and myopathy with hyperthyroidism.[114]

Numerous treatment modalities have been reported in the literature, but often with inconsistent results, frequent relapses, and potentially serious side effects including intralesional corticosteroids, melphalan, phototherapy, systemic retinoids, plasmapheresis, and autologous hematopoietic stem cell transplantation. Improvement with IVIG[115] or thalidomide has also been reported.[116] Overall, scleromyxedema tends to follow a chronic and progressive course and patients may ultimately succumb from systemic complications.

PANNICULITIS AND FASCIITIS ASSOCIATED WITH INTERNAL MALIGNANCY
Pancreatic Panniculitis

Pancreatic panniculitis is an uncommon condition affecting 2% to 3% of patients with pancreatic disorders.[117] Clinically, it presents with ill-defined, tender, erythematous to red-brown subcutaneous nodules that may spontaneously ulcerate and drain an oily brown viscous substance.[118] The lesions are typically found on the distal lower extremities; however, in pancreatic panniculitis associated with pancreatic carcinoma, they may be found in other areas of the body as well.[118] Pancreatic panniculitis associated with pancreatic tumor, eosinophilia, and polyarthritis is known as the Schmid triad and is associated with a poor prognosis.[119]

Although pancreatic panniculitis is most commonly associated with acute and chronic pancreatitis of various causes, there are numerous reports of this condition developing in association with pancreatic neoplasia. Associated neoplasms include acinar carcinoma,[120–123] neuroendocrine carcinoma,[124] and acinar cell cystadenocarcinoma.[119] Although comprising less than 2% of all pancreatic neoplasms, acinar cell carcinoma is associated with pancreatic panniculitis in 10% of cases, making it the most commonly associated neoplasm.[123] Pancreatic panniculitis has also been reported in a case of pancreatic metastasis from gastric carcinoma.[125] The onset of pancreatic panniculitis relative to the diagnosis of the underlying neoplasm is variable; however, it has been reported to predate discovery of the pancreatic neoplasm by up to several months.[118,125–127] Pancreatic panniculitis may suggest a more aggressive course of the underlying neoplasm.[127]

The mainstay of treatment of pancreatic panniculitis is removal of the underlying neoplasm, which has been reported in some cases to completely resolve the panniculitis.[120,128] Octreotide, a somatostatin analogue, has been reported to prevent spread of panniculitis in patients who are not candidates for tumor resection.[129,130]

Neutrophilic Panniculitis in Myeloproliferative Disorders

In 1982, Leibowitz and colleagues[131] described a 34-year-old woman with a variant of Sweet's syndrome extending into the subcutaneous fat who was found to have a dyserythropoiesis on bone marrow biopsy. This case was the first description of neutrophilic panniculitis associated with an underlying malignancy. Since then, there have been sporadic case reports of neutrophilic panniculitis associated with several malignancies, most commonly myeloproliferative disorders.[132,133] Clinically, the lesions are tender, erythematous plaques or nodules that favor the limbs.[133] Characteristically, patients are systemically ill, often with fever, pain, and arthralgia.[133] The incidence of panniculitis in patients with myeloproliferative disorder is unknown; however, it is rare. One study of 2357 patients with multiple myeloma, in which an associated neutrophilic panniculitis was reported, revealed only 1 patient with a skin biopsy revealing panniculitis.[134]

Myeloproliferative disorders associated with neutrophilic panniculitis include myelodysplastic syndrome, acute myeloid leukemia, multiple myeloma, and dyserythropoiesis.[132,133] More recently, there have been case reports of neutrophilic panniculitis associated with metastasis from prostate cancer and breast cancer.[135,136] Panniculitis has been reported as the presenting sign of hematological malignancy.[131,137] It has also developed on initiation of certain medications in the setting of hematologic malignancy, specifically all-transretinoic acid in a patient with acute promyelocytic leukemia, imatinib, and subsequently dasatinib, in a single patient with chronic myelogenous leukemia.[138,139]

The existence of neutrophilic lobular panniculitis as a distinct histopathologic entity has been challenged and may be a presentation of subcutaneous Sweet's syndrome.[140] High-dose corticosteroids have resulted in rapid clinical improvement of the panniculitis; other antineutrophilic agents such as dapsone and colchicine have also been tried with success.[133]

Palmar Fasciitis and Polyarthritis

Palmar fasciitis and polyarthritis syndrome (PFPAS) was first recognized as a distinct entity by Medsger and colleagues[141] in 1982, when they presented a case series of 6 patients with painful hand contractures and polyarthritis who were found to have ovarian carcinomas. Since then, more than 40 cases of this syndrome have been published in the literature. In most cases, the hands develop diffuse painful swelling and stiffness with subsequent nodular thickening of the palmar fascia.[142] Skin surface changes may include erythema at the periphery of the palms or indurated, reticular erythema over the central palm.[143] Synovitis and polyarthritis favor the small joints of the hand; joint involvement at other locations, such as the shoulders, elbows, wrists, knees, ankles, and feet, has been reported but symptoms are typically less severe.[142,144,145] Severity of symptoms can range from mild to completely disabling.[145]

The most common neoplasm associated with PFPAS is ovarian carcinoma; however, many associated malignancies have been reported, including pancreas, lung, colon, prostate, breast, hepatocellular, renal pelvis, uterine cervix, gastric, gastroesophageal, Hodgkin disease, multiple myeloma, and chronic myelogenous leukemia.[144,146] Several benign conditions have also been associated and, in some cases, no underlying cause has been found.[146] Typically PFPAS develops before diagnosis of the underlying malignancy with reported onset as early as 23 months before diagnosis.[141,147] In addition, PFPAS has occurred on treatment of gastroesophageal cancer with a matrix metalloproteinase inhibitor.[148]

Radiographs of the affected joints are typically unremarkable except for variable periarticular demineralization and soft tissue swelling.[142,145] Symptoms of polyarthritis and pain have been reported to improve with treatment of the underlying malignancy, but palmar fibrosis and resulting contractures tend to be persistent.[144,147] Systemic glucocorticoids have been of modest benefit for symptom relief in several cases but are usually ineffective.[144,146,148,149]

Eosinophilic Fasciitis and Fasciitis-Panniculitis Syndrome

In 1975, Shulman[150] reported a syndrome involving fibrotic thickening of the subcutaneous fat and fascia with variable infiltration of eosinophils and/or peripheral eosinophilia, which was subsequently termed eosinophilic fasciitis. In 1992, Naschitz and colleagues[151] described a series of patients with similar clinical and histologic features to eosinophilic fasciitis; however, they noted that peripheral and tissue eosinophilia were inconsistent findings. They coined the term fasciitis-panniculitis syndrome (FPS), which included eosinophilic fasciitis in addition to other entities involving subcutaneous-fascial fibrosis such as lipodermatosclerosis, chronic graft-versus-host disease, postirradiation injury, and others. Clinically, eosinophilic fasciitis and FPS are characterized by 1 or more areas of sleevelike and/or plaquelike swelling or induration of the skin.[152] The lower extremity is most commonly affected; however, neck, forearm, wrist, and generalized involvement have been reported.[152] Eosinophilic fasciitis is known to display a progression from edema of the affected extremities, then to hyperpigmented peau d'orange skin, then to woody induration with skin tightness.[153] Extracutaneous manifestations occur in 5% to 15% of patients and may include arthritis, hepatitis, pericarditis, colitis, pleuritis, pulmonary fibrosis, esophageal disturbances, thyroid disease, Sjögren syndrome, and Raynaud phenomenon.[154]

The true incidence of malignancy-associated eosinophilic fasciitis and FPS is unknown, although Naschitz and colleagues[154] reported 3 patients in an 8-year period at an institution serving more than 150,000 patients in Israel. Only a small percentage of eosinophilic fasciitis and FPS is associated with malignancy: 4 patients in a series of 52 and 3 patients in a series of 19, respectively.[154,155] Hematologic malignancies are most commonly associated with eosinophilic fasciitis and FPS, but solid organ tumors have also been reported. Specifically, malignancies associated with eosinophilic fasciitis include myeloproliferative disorder, myelomonocytic leukemia, chronic lymphocytic leukemia, porphyria cutanea tarda, Hodgkin disease, immunoblastic lymphoma, T-cell lymphoma, breast carcinoma, and colorectal carcinoma.[155–158] Associations with FPS include myelomonocytic leukemia, chronic lymphocytic leukemia, myeloproliferative disorder, Hodgkin disease, T-cell lymphoma, breast carcinoma, prostate carcinoma, gastric adenocarcinoma, and pancreatic carcinoma.[154,159–161] The onset of FPS typically precedes the onset of hematological malignancy from months to 3.5 years; however, timing of onset of associated solid organ malignancies was more variable.[154,158,160]

Although idiopathic eosinophilic fasciitis and FPS are usually corticosteroid responsive, paraneoplastic eosinophilic fasciitis and FPS are not consistently improved with steroids.[153,156] Eosinophilic fasciitis and FPS may remit after successful treatment of the neoplasm.[153,156,158,160]

SUMMARY

The skin changes outlined in this article can be important clues to an underlying malignancy. Paraneoplastic dermatoses are skin disorders associated with an underlying neoplasm and whose course parallels that of the neoplasm. Recognizing these skin presentations leads to early diagnosis and management of the underlying malignancy. Effective treatment of the associated neoplasm often leads to improvement of the cutaneous manifestations and should be the primary focus of each patient's management.

REFERENCES

1. Clarke J. Malignant acanthosis nigricans. Clin Exp Dermatol 1977;2(2):167–70.
2. Cohen PR, Grossman ME, Almeida L, et al. Tripe palms and malignancy. J Clin Oncol 1989;7(5):669–78.
3. Khaled A, Abdallah MB, Tekaya R, et al. Tripe palms with oligoarthritis, two rare paraneoplastic syndromes heralding a small cell lung cancer. J Eur Acad Dermatol Venereol 2009;23(5):579–80.
4. Breathnach SM, Wells GC. Acanthosis palmaris: tripe palms. A distinctive pattern of palmar keratoderma frequently associated with internal malignancy. Clin Exp Dermatol 1980;5(2):181–9.
5. Cohen PR, Grossman ME, Silvers DN, et al. Tripe palms and cancer. Clin Dermatol 1993;11(1):165–73.
6. Cohen PR. Hypertrophic pulmonary osteoarthropathy and tripe palms in a man with squamous cell carcinoma of the larynx and lung. Report of a case and

review of cutaneous paraneoplastic syndromes associated with laryngeal and lung malignancies. Am J Clin Oncol 1993;16(3):268–76.

7. Moore RL, Devere TS. Epidermal manifestations of internal malignancy. Dermatol Clin 2008;26(1):17–29, vii.

8. Schwartz RA. Acanthosis nigricans. J Am Acad Dermatol 1994;31(1):1–19 [quiz: 20–2].

9. Lo WL, Wong CK. Tripe palms: a significant cutaneous sign of internal malignancy. Dermatology 1992;185(2):151–3.

10. Hazen PG, Carney JF, Walker AE, et al. Acanthosis nigricans presenting as hyperkeratosis of the palms and soles. J Am Acad Dermatol 1979;1(6):541–4.

11. Gorisek B, Krajnc I, Rems D, et al. Malignant acanthosis nigricans and tripe palms in a patient with endometrial adenocarcinoma–a case report and review of literature. Gynecol Oncol 1997;65(3):539–42.

12. Sedano HO, Gorlin RJ. Acanthosis nigricans. Oral Surg Oral Med Oral Pathol 1987;63(4):462–7.

13. Cohen PR. Cutaneous paraneoplastic syndromes. Am Fam Physician 1994; 50(6):1273–82.

14. Brown J, Winkelmann RK. Acanthosis nigricans: a study of 90 cases. Medicine (Baltimore) 1968;47(1):33–51.

15. Curth HO. Acanthosis nigricans and its association with cancer. Arch Derm Syphilol 1948;57(2):158–70.

16. Weger W, Ginter-Hanselmayer G, Hammer HF, et al. Florid cutaneous papillomatosis with acanthosis nigricans in a patient with carcinomas of the lung and prostate. J Am Acad Dermatol 2007;57(5):907–8.

17. Krawczyk M, Mykala-Ciesla J, Kolodziej-Jaskula A. Acanthosis nigricans as a paraneoplastic syndrome. Case reports and review of literature. Pol Arch Med Wewn 2009;119(3):180–3.

18. Kaminska-Winciorek G, Brzezinska-Wcislo L, Lis-Swiety A, et al. Paraneoplastic type of acanthosis nigricans in patient with hepatocellular carcinoma. Adv Med Sci 2007;52:254–6.

19. Janier M, Blanchet-Bardon C, Bonvalet D, et al. Malignant acanthosis nigricans associated with non-Hodgkin's lymphoma. Report of 2 cases. Dermatologica 1988;176(3):133–7.

20. Schwartz RA. Acanthosis nigricans, florid cutaneous papillomatosis and the sign of Leser-Trelat. Cutis 1981;28(3):319–22, 326–7, 330–1 passim.

21. Bersaques DJ. Sign of Leser-Trelat [letter]. J Am Acad Dermatol Clin 1985;12:724.

22. Hollander EV. Beitrage zur Fruhdiagnose des Darmcarcinoms (Hereditatsverhaltnisse und Hautveranderungen.). Dtsch Med Wochenschr 1900;26:483–5.

23. Holdiness MR. On the classification of the sign of Leser-Trelat. J Am Acad Dermatol 1988;19(4):754–7.

24. Dantzig PI. Sign of Leser-Trelat. Arch Dermatol 1973;108(5):700–1.

25. Ellis DL, Yates RA. Sign of Leser-Trelat. Clin Dermatol 1993;11(1):141–8.

26. Barron LA, Prendiville JS. The sign of Leser-Trelat in a young woman with osteogenic sarcoma. J Am Acad Dermatol 1992;26(2 Pt 2):344–7.

27. Bazex A, Griffiths A. Acrokeratosis paraneoplastica–a new cutaneous marker of malignancy. Br J Dermatol 1980;103(3):301–6.

28. Bolognia JL, Brewer YP, Cooper DL. Bazex syndrome (acrokeratosis paraneoplastica). An analytic review. Medicine (Baltimore) 1991;70(4):269–80.

29. Gill D, Fergin P, Kelly J. Bullous lesions in Bazex syndrome and successful treatment with oral psoralen phototherapy. Australas J Dermatol 2001;42(4): 278–80.

30. Pecora AL, Landsman L, Imgrund SP, et al. Acrokeratosis paraneoplastica (Bazex' syndrome). Report of a case and review of the literature. Arch Dermatol 1983;119(10):820–6.
31. Jacobsen FK, Abildtrup N, Laursen SO, et al. Acrokeratosis paraneoplastica (Bazex' syndrome). Arch Dermatol 1984;120(4):502–4.
32. Sarkar B, Knecht R, Sarkar C, et al. Bazex syndrome (acrokeratosis paraneoplastica). Eur Arch Otorhinolaryngol 1998;255(4):205–10.
33. da Rosa AC, Pinto GM, Bortoluzzi JS, et al. Three simultaneous paraneoplastic manifestations (ichthyosis acquisita, Bazex syndrome, and Leser-Trelat sign) with prostate adenocarcinoma. J Am Acad Dermatol 2009;61(3):538–40.
34. Esteve E, Serpier H, Cambie MP, et al. Bazex paraneoplastic acrokeratosis. Treatment with acitretin. Ann Dermatol Venereol 1995;122(1-2):26–9 [in French].
35. Schwartz RA, Williams ML. Acquired ichthyosis: a marker for internal disease. Am Fam Physician 1984;29(2):181–4.
36. Aram H. Acquired ichthyosis and related conditions. Int J Dermatol 1984;23(7):458–61.
37. Ronchese F. Ichthyosiform atrophy of the skin in Hodgkin's disease. Arch Derm Syphilol 1943;47:778–81.
38. Tlacuilo-Parra JA, Guevara-Gutierrez E, Salazar-Paramo M. Acquired ichthyosis associated with systemic lupus erythematosus. Lupus 2004;13(4):270–3.
39. Okulicz JF, Schwartz RA. Hereditary and acquired ichthyosis vulgaris. Int J Dermatol 2003;42(2):95–8.
40. Van Dijk E. Ichthyosiform atrophy of the skin associated with internal malignant diseases. Dermatologica 1963;127:413–28.
41. Kurzrock R, Cohen PR. Mucocutaneous paraneoplastic manifestations of hematologic malignancies. Am J Med 1995;99(2):207–16.
42. Levy O, Tishler M. Acquired ichthyosis as the primary manifestation of renal cell carcinoma. Isr Med Assoc J 2009;11(2):121–2.
43. Lucker GP, Steijlen PM. Acrokeratosis paraneoplastica (Bazex syndrome) occurring with acquired ichthyosis in Hodgkin's disease. Br J Dermatol 1995;133(2):322–5.
44. Penven K, Verneuil L, Dompmartin A, et al. [An association of paraneoplastic syndromes in a patient]. Ann Dermatol Venereol 2002;129(8-9):1042–5 [in French].
45. Roselino AM, Souza CS, Andrade JM, et al. Dermatomyositis and acquired ichthyosis as paraneoplastic manifestations of ovarian tumor. Int J Dermatol 1997;36(8):611–4.
46. Rizos E, Milionis HJ, Pavlidis N, et al. Acquired ichthyosis: a paraneoplastic skin manifestation of Hodgkin's disease. Lancet Oncol 2002;3(12):727.
47. Griffin LJ, Massa MC. Acquired ichthyosis and pityriasis rotunda. Clin Dermatol 1993;11(1):27–32.
48. Ameen M, Chopra S, Darvay A, et al. Erythema gyratum repens and acquired ichthyosis associated with transitional cell carcinoma of the kidney. Clin Exp Dermatol 2001;26(6):510–2.
49. Gammel JA. Erythema gyratum repens; skin manifestations in patient with carcinoma of breast. AMA Arch Derm Syphilol 1952;66(4):494–505.
50. Boyd AS, Neldner KH, Menter A. Erythema gyratum repens: a paraneoplastic eruption. J Am Acad Dermatol 1992;26(5 Pt 1):757–62.
51. Almaani N, Robson A, Sarkany R, et al. Erythema gyratum repens associated with pityriasis rubra pilaris. Clin Exp Dermatol 2011;36(2):161–4.
52. Stone SP, Buescher LS. Life-threatening paraneoplastic cutaneous syndromes. Clin Dermatol 2005;23(3):301–6.

53. Eubanks LE, McBurney E, Reed R. Erythema gyratum repens. Am J Med Sci 2001;321(5):302–5.
54. Kwatra A, McDonald RE, Corriere JN Jr. Erythema gyratum repens in association with renal cell carcinoma. J Urol 1998;159(6):2077.
55. Skolnick M, Mainman ER. Erythema gyratum repens with metastatic adenocarcinoma. Arch Dermatol 1975;111(2):227–9.
56. Becker SW, Kahn D, Rothman S. Cutaneous manifestations of internal malignant tumors. Arch Derm Syphilol 1942;45:1069–80.
57. McGavran MH, Unger RH, Recant L, et al. A glucagon-secreting alpha-cell carcinoma of the pancreas. N Engl J Med 1966;274(25):1408–13.
58. Wilkinson DS. Necrolytic migratory erythema with pancreatic carcinoma. Proc R Soc Med 1971;64(12):1197–8.
59. Wilkinson DS. Necrolytic migratory erythema with carcinoma of the pancreas. Trans St Johns Hosp Dermatol Soc 1973;59(2):244–50.
60. Wermers RA, Fatourechi V, Wynne AG, et al. The glucagonoma syndrome. Clinical and pathologic features in 21 patients. Medicine (Baltimore) 1996;75(2):53–63.
61. van Beek AP, de Haas ER, van Vloten WA, et al. The glucagonoma syndrome and necrolytic migratory erythema: a clinical review. Eur J Endocrinol 2004;151(5):531–7.
62. Adam DN, Cohen PD, Ghazarian D. Necrolytic migratory erythema: case report and clinical review. J Cutan Med Surg 2003;7(4):333–8.
63. Shi W, Liao W, Mei X, et al. Necrolytic migratory erythema associated with glucagonoma syndrome. J Clin Oncol 2010;28(20):e329–31.
64. Mallinson CN, Bloom SR, Warin AP, et al. A glucagonoma syndrome. Lancet 1974;2(7871):1–5.
65. Frankton S, Bloom SR. Gastrointestinal endocrine tumours. Glucagonomas. Baillieres Clin Gastroenterol 1996;10(4):697–705.
66. Tierney EP, Badger J. Etiology and pathogenesis of necrolytic migratory erythema: review of the literature. MedGenMed 2004;6(3):4.
67. Kheir SM, Omura EF, Grizzle WE, et al. Histologic variation in the skin lesions of the glucagonoma syndrome. Am J Surg Pathol 1986;10(7):445–53.
68. Soga J, Yakuwa Y. Glucagonomas/diabetico-dermatogenic syndrome (DDS): a statistical evaluation of 407 reported cases. J Hepatobiliary Pancreat Surg 1998;5(3):312–9.
69. Mullans EA, Cohen PR. Iatrogenic necrolytic migratory erythema: a case report and review of nonglucagonoma-associated necrolytic migratory erythema. J Am Acad Dermatol 1998;38(5 Pt 2):866–73.
70. Johnson SM, Smoller BR, Lamps LW, et al. Necrolytic migratory erythema as the only presenting sign of a glucagonoma. J Am Acad Dermatol 2003;49(2):325–8.
71. Bewley AP, Ross JS, Bunker CB, et al. Successful treatment of a patient with octreotide-resistant necrolytic migratory erythema. Br J Dermatol 1996;134(6):1101–4.
72. Vandersteen PR, Scheithauer BW. Glucagonoma syndrome. A clinicopathologic, immunocytochemical, and ultrastructural study. J Am Acad Dermatol 1985;12(6):1032–9.
73. Stertz G. Polymyositis. Berl Klin Wochenshr 1916;53:489.
74. Zahr ZA, Baer AN. Malignancy in myositis. Curr Rheumatol Rep 2011;13(3):208–15.
75. Callen JP, Wortmann RL. Dermatomyositis. Clin Dermatol 2006;24(5):363–73.
76. Targoff IN, Mamyrova G, Trieu EP, et al. A novel autoantibody to a 155-kd protein is associated with dermatomyositis. Arthritis Rheum 2006;54(11):3682–9.

77. Callen JP. When and how should the patient with dermatomyositis or amyopathic dermatomyositis be assessed for possible cancer? Arch Dermatol 2002;138(7):969–71.

78. Wakata N, Kurihara T, Saito E, et al. Polymyositis and dermatomyositis associated with malignancy: a 30-year retrospective study. Int J Dermatol 2002; 41(11):729–34.

79. Fardet L, Dupuy A, Gain M, et al. Factors associated with underlying malignancy in a retrospective cohort of 121 patients with dermatomyositis. Medicine (Baltimore) 2009;88(2):91–7.

80. Kaji K, Fujimoto M, Hasegawa M, et al. Identification of a novel autoantibody reactive with 155 and 140 kDa nuclear proteins in patients with dermatomyositis: an association with malignancy. Rheumatology (Oxford) 2007;46(1):25–8.

81. Andras C, Ponyi A, Constantin T, et al. Dermatomyositis and polymyositis associated with malignancy: a 21-year retrospective study. J Rheumatol 2008;35(3): 438–44.

82. Callen JP. Dermatomyositis: diagnosis, evaluation and management. Minerva Med 2002;93(3):157–67.

83. Anhalt GJ, Kim S, Stanley JR, et al. Paraneoplastic pemphigus – an autoimmune mucocutaneous disease associated with neoplasia. N Engl J Med 1990;323: 1729–35.

84. Anhalt GJ. Paraneoplastic pemphigus. J Investig Dermatol Symp Proc 2004; 9(1):29–33.

85. Chung VQ, Moschella SL, Zembowicz A, et al. Clinical and pathologic findings of paraneoplastic dermatoses. J Am Acad Dermatol 2006;54(5):745–62, 86.

86. Allen CM, Camisa C. Paraneoplastic pemphigus: a review of the literature. Oral Dis 2000;6:208–14.

87. Nikolskaia OV, Nousari CH, Anhalt GJ. Paraneoplastic pemphigus in association with Castleman's disease. Br J Dermatol 2003;149:1143–51.

88. Wade MS, Black MM. Paraneoplastic pemphigus: a brief update. Australas J Dermatol 2005;46:1–8.

89. Maldonado R, Pittelkow MR, Ryu JH. Constrictive bronchiolitis associated with paraneoplastic autoimmune multiorgan syndrome. Respirology 2009;14:129–33.

90. Sweet RD. An acute febrile neutrophilic dermatosis. Br J Dermatol 1964;76: 349–56.

91. Moschella SL, Davis MD. Neutrophilic dermatoses. In: Bolognia J, Jorizzo JL, Rapini RP, editors. Dermatology. London, New York: Mosby; 2008. p. 381.

92. Neoh CY, Tan AW, Mg SK. Sweet's syndrome: a spectrum of unusual clinical presentations and associations. Br J Dermatol 2007;156:480–5.

93. Cohen PR, Talpaz M, Kurzrock R. Malignancy-associated Sweet's syndrome: review of the world literature. J Clin Oncol 1988;6(12):1887–97.

94. Cohen PR, Kurzrock R. Sweet's syndrome revisited: a review of disease concepts. Int J Dermatol 2003;42(10):761–78.

95. Bourke JF, Keohane S, Long CC, et al. Sweet's syndrome and malignancy in the UK. Br J Dermatol 1997;137(4):609–13.

96. Cohen PR. Sweet's syndrome–a comprehensive review of an acute febrile neutrophilic dermatosis. Orphanet J Rare Dis 2007;26(2):34.

97. Goodman WT, Barrett TL. Histocytoses. In: Bolognia J, Jorizzo JL, Rapini RP, editors. Dermatology. London, New York: Mosby; 2008. p. 1404 p. 1406.

98. Ugurlu S, Bartley GB, Gibson LE. Necrobiotic xanthogranuloma: long-term outcome of ocular and systemic involvement. Am J Ophthalmol 2000;129(5): 651–6.

99. Mehregan DA, Winkelmann RK. Necrobiotic xanthogranuloma. Arch Dermatol 1992;128(1):94–100.
100. Goltz RW, Laymon CW. Multicentric reticulohistiocytosis of the skin and synovia; reticulohistiocytoma or ganglioneuroma. AMA Arch Derm Syphilol 1954;69(6): 717–31.
101. Luz FB, Gaspar TA, Kalil-Gaspar N, et al. Multicentric reticulohistiocytosis. J Eur Acad Dermatol Venereol 2001;15(6):524–31.
102. Gravallese EM, Goldring SR. Cellular mechanisms and the role of cytokines in bone erosions in rheumatoid arthritis. Arthritis Rheum 2000;43:2143–51.
103. Codriansky KA, Rünger TM, Bhawan J, et al. Multicentric reticulohistiocytosis: a systemic osteoclastic disease? Arthritis Rheum 2008;59(3):444–8.
104. Rentsch JL, Martin EM, Harrison LC, et al. Prolonged response of multicentric reticulohistiocytosis to low dose methotrexate. J Rheumatol 1998;25(5):1012–5.
105. Gorman JD, Danning C, Schumacher HR, et al. Multicentric reticulohistiocytosis: case report with immunohistochemical analysis and literature review. Arthritis Rheum 2000;43(4):930–8.
106. De Knop KJ, Aerts NE, Ebo DG, et al. Multicentric reticulohistiocytosis associated arthritis responding to anti-TNF and methotrexate. Acta Clin Belg 2011; 66(1):66–9.
107. Goto H, Inaba M, Kobayashi K, et al. Successful treatment of multicentric reticulohistiocytosis with alendronate: evidence for a direct effect of bisphosphonate on histiocytes. Arthritis Rheum 2003;48(12):3538–41.
108. Satoh M, Oyama N, Yamada H, et al. Treatment trial of multicentric reticulohistiocytosis with a combination of predonisolone, methotrexate and alendronate. J Dermatol 2008;35(3):168–71.
109. Rongioletti F, Rebora A. Updated classification of papular mucinosis, lichen myxedematosus, and scleromyxedema. J Am Acad Dermatol 2001;44(2): 273–81.
110. Rongioletti F. Lichen myxedematosus (papular mucinosis): new concepts and perspectives for an old disease. Semin Cutan Med Surg 2006;25(2): 100–4.
111. Gabriel SE, Perry HO, Oleson GB, et al. Scleromyxedema: a scleroderma-like disorder with systemic manifestations. Medicine 1988;67(1):58–65.
112. Kitamura W, Matsuoka Y, Miyagawa S, et al. Immunochemical analysis of the monoclonal paraprotein in scleromyxedema. J Invest Dermatol 1978;70(6): 305–8.
113. Launay D, Hatron PY, Delaporte E, et al. Scleromyxedema (lichen myxedematosus) associated with dermatomyositis. Br J Dermatol 2001;144(2):359–62.
114. Van Linthoudt D, Schumacher HR Jr, Algeo S, et al. Scleromyxedema with myopathy and hyperthyroidism. J Rheumatol 1996;23(7):1299–301.
115. Lister RK, Jolles S, Whittaker S, et al. Scleromyxedema: response to high-dose intravenous immunoglobulin (hdIVIg). J Am Acad Dermatol 2000;43(2, part 2): 403–8.
116. Sansbury JC, Cocuroccia B, Jorizzo JL, et al. Treatment of recalcitrant scleromyxedema with thalidomide in 3 patients. J Am Acad Dermatol 2004;51(1): 126–31.
117. Potts DE, Mass MF, Iseman MD. Syndrome and pancreatic disease, subcutaneous fat necrosis and polyserositis. Case report and review of literature. Am J Med 1975;58(3):417–23.
110. García-Romero D, Vanaclocha F. Pancreatic panniculitis. Dermatol Clin 2008; 26(4):465–70, vi.

119. Beltraminelli HS, Buechner SA, Häusermann P. Pancreatic panniculitis in a patient with an acinar cell cystadenocarcinoma of the pancreas. Dermatology 2004;208(3):265–7.

120. Moro M, Moletta L, Blandamura S, et al. Acinar cell carcinoma of the pancreas associated with subcutaneous panniculitis. JOP 2011;12(3):292–6.

121. Poelman SM, Nguyen K. Pancreatic panniculitis associated with acinar cell pancreatic carcinoma. J Cutan Med Surg 2008;12(1):38–42.

122. Heykarts B, Anseeuw M, Degreef H. Panniculitis caused by acinous pancreatic carcinoma. Dermatology 1999;198(2):182–3.

123. Klimstra DS, Heffess CS, Oertel JE, et al. Acinar cell carcinoma of the pancreas. A clinicopathologic study of 28 cases. Am J Surg Pathol 1992;16(9):815–37.

124. Martin SK, Agarwal G, Lynch GR. Subcutaneous fat necrosis as the presenting feature of a pancreatic carcinoma: the challenge of differentiating endocrine and acinar pancreatic neoplasms. Pancreas 2009;38(2):219–22.

125. Beyazıt H, Aydin O, Demirkesen C, et al. Pancreatic panniculitis as the first manifestation of the pancreatic involvement during the course of a gastric adenocarcinoma. Med Oncol 2011;28(1):137–9.

126. Gandhi RK, Bechtel M, Peters S, et al. Pancreatic panniculitis in a patient with BRCA2 mutation and metastatic pancreatic adenocarcinoma. Int J Dermatol 2010;49(12):1419–20.

127. Marsh Rde W, Hagler KT, Carag HR, et al. Pancreatic panniculitis. Eur J Surg Oncol 2005;31(10):1213–5.

128. Kuerer H, Shim H, Pertsemlidis D, et al. Functioning pancreatic acinar cell carcinoma: immunohistochemical and ultrastructural analyses. Am J Clin Oncol 1997;20(1):101–7.

129. Hudson-peacock MJ, Regnard CF, Farr PM. Liquefying panniculitis associated with acinous carcinoma of the pancreas responding to octreotide. J R Soc Med 1994;87(6):361–2.

130. Durden FM, Variyam E, Chren MM. Fat necrosis with features of erythema nodosum in a patient with metastatic pancreatic carcinoma. Int J Dermatol 1996; 35(1):39–41.

131. Leibowitz MR, Rippey JJ, Bezwoda WR, et al. Unusual aspects of febrile neutrophilic dermatosis (Sweet's syndrome). Case reports. S Afr Med J 1982;62(11): 375–8.

132. Chen HC, Kao WY, Chang DM, et al. Neutrophilic panniculitis with myelodysplastic syndromes presenting as pustulosis: case report and review of the literature. Am J Hematol 2004;76(1):61–5.

133. Sutra-Loubet C, Carlotti A, Guillemette J, et al. Neutrophilic panniculitis. J Am Acad Dermatol 2004;50(2):280–5.

134. Bayer-garner IB, Smoller BR. The spectrum of cutaneous disease in multiple myeloma. J Am Acad Dermatol 2003;48(4):497–507.

135. Kim J, Choi YJ, Oh SH, et al. A case of Sweet's panniculitis associated with spinal metastasis from prostate cancer. Ann Dermatol 2010;22(4):478–81.

136. Teng JM, Draper BK, Boyd AS. Sweet's panniculitis associated with metastatic breast cancer. J Am Acad Dermatol 2007;56(Suppl 2):S61–2.

137. Hendrickx G, Nooijen P, De Raeve L. Panniculitis as the presenting sign of a myelodysplastic syndrome in an adolescent boy. Pediatr Dermatol 2009; 26(2):219–22.

138. Jagdeo J, Campbell R, Long T, et al. Sweet's syndrome–like neutrophilic lobular panniculitis associated with all-trans-retinoic acid chemotherapy in a patient with acute promyelocytic leukemia. J Am Acad Dermatol 2007;56(4):690–3.

139. de Masson A, Bouvresse S, Clérici T, et al. [Recurrent neutrophilic panniculitis in a patient with chronic myelogenous leukaemia treated with imatinib mesilate and dasatinib]. Ann Dermatol Venereol 2011;138(2):135–9 [in French].

140. Cohen PR. Subcutaneous Sweet's syndrome: a variant of acute febrile neutrophilic dermatosis that is included in the histopathologic differential diagnosis of neutrophilic panniculitis. J Am Acad Dermatol 2005;52(5): 927–8.

141. Medsger TA, Dixon JA, Garwood VF. Palmar fasciitis and polyarthritis associated with ovarian carcinoma. Ann Intern Med 1982;96(4):424–31.

142. Eekhoff EM, van der Lubbe PA, Breedveld FC. Flexion contractures associated with a malignant neoplasm: 'A paraneoplastic syndrome?'. Clin Rheumatol 1998;17(2):157–9.

143. Preda VA, Frederiksen P, Kossard S. Indurated reticulate palmar erythema as a sign of paraneoplastic palmar fasciitis and polyarthritis syndrome. Australas J Dermatol 2009;50(3):198–201.

144. Clarke LL, Kennedy CT, Hollingworth P. Palmar fasciitis and polyarthritis syndrome associated with transitional cell carcinoma of the bladder. J Am Acad Dermatol 2011;64(6):1159–1163, e2.

145. Krishna K, Yacoub A, Hutchins LF, et al. Palmar fasciitis with polyarthritis syndrome in a patient with breast cancer. Clin Rheumatol 2011;30(4):569–72.

146. Sung YK, Park MH, Yoo DH. Idiopathic palmar fasciitis with polyarthritis syndrome. J Korean Med Sci 2006;21(6):1128–32.

147. Martorell EA, Murray PM, Peterson JJ, et al. Palmar fasciitis and arthritis syndrome associated with metastatic ovarian carcinoma: a report of four cases. J Hand Surg Am 2004;29(4):654–60.

148. Virik K, Lynch KP, Harper P. Gastroesophageal cancer, palmar fasciitis and a matrix metalloproteinase inhibitor. Intern Med J 2002;32(1-2):50–1.

149. Willemse PH, Mulder NH, van de Tempel HJ, et al. Palmar fasciitis and arthritis in a patient with an extraovarian adenocarcinoma of the coelomic epithelium. Ann Rheum Dis 1991;50(1):53–4.

150. Shulman LE. Diffuse fasciitis with eosinophilia: a new syndrome? Trans Assoc Am Physicians 1975;88:70–86.

151. Naschitz JE, Yeshurun D, Zuckerman E, et al. The fasciitis-panniculitis syndrome: clinical spectrum and response to cimetidine. Semin Arthritis Rheum 1992;21(4):211–20.

152. Naschitz JE, Boss JH, Misselevich I, et al. The fasciitis-panniculitis syndromes. Clinical and pathologic features. Medicine (Baltimore) 1996; 75(1):6–16.

153. Bischoff L, Derk CT. Eosinophilic fasciitis: demographics, disease pattern and response to treatment: report of 12 cases and review of the literature. Int J Dermatol 2008;47(1):29–35.

154. Naschitz JE, Yeshurun D, Zuckerman E, et al. Cancer-associated fasciitis panniculitis. Cancer 1994;73(1):231–5.

155. Lakhanpal S, Ginsburg WW, Michet CJ, et al. Eosinophilic fasciitis: clinical spectrum and therapeutic response in 52 cases. Semin Arthritis Rheum 1988;17(4): 221–31.

156. Naschitz JE, Misselevich I, Rosner I, et al. Lymph-node-based malignant lymphoma and reactive lymphadenopathy in eosinophilic fasciitis. Am J Med Sci 1999;318(5):343–9.

157. Jacob SE, Lodha R, Cohen JJ, et al. Paraneoplastic eosinophilic fasciitis: a case report. Rheumatol Int 2003;23(5):262–4.

158. Philpott H, Hissaria P, Warrren L, et al. Eosinophilic fasciitis as a paraneoplastic phenomenon associated with metastatic colorectal carcinoma. Australas J Dermatol 2008;49(1):27–9.

159. Ido T, Kiyohara T, Sawai T, et al. Fasciitis-panniculitis syndrome and advanced gastric adenocarcinoma in association with antibodies to single-stranded DNA. Br J Dermatol 2006;155(3):640–1.

160. Dinakar P, Höke A. Paraneoplastic fasciitis-panniculitis syndrome: a neurological point of view. Nat Clin Pract Neurol 2009;5(2):113–7.

161. Kuempers P, Köhler L, Pertschy S, et al. Unilateral fasciitis of the lower leg: a paraneoplastic manifestation of an occult pancreatic tumor. J Clin Rheumatol 2006; 12(3):139–41.

Neoplastic and Paraneoplastic Vasculitis, Vasculopathy, and Hypercoagulability

Hyon Ju Park, MD[a,b], Prabha Ranganathan, MD, MS[a,b],*

KEYWORDS

- Neoplastic • Paraneoplastic • Vasculitis • Vasculopathy
- Hypercoagulability

Rheumatologists are often consulted regarding both typical and atypical vasculitides, vasculopathies, and hypercoagulability. It is important to keep in mind that all of these can come from neoplastic or paraneoplastic causes. In these cases, the treatment must focus on treating the underlying malignancy rather than aggressive immunosuppression. This article focuses on reported cases, pathophysiologic mechanisms, and lessons that can learned from the literature regarding neoplastic and paraneoplastic vasculitides, vasculopathies, and hypercoagulability.

Currently, the literature regarding malignancy-related vasculitides, vasculopathies, and hypercoagulability mostly comprises case reports. Some reports are on cases in which the paraneoplastic phenomenon precedes the diagnosis of malignancies by years.[1,2] However, there are many case-series and registry data suggesting that certain vasculitides, vasculopathies, and hypercoagulability states (eg, antiphospholipid syndrome) may increase the risk of malignancy.[3,4] Medications commonly used in treating these vascular syndromes have also been reported to increase the risk of malignancy.[5,6] There are also reports of specific chemotherapy drugs causing cutaneous vasculitis.[7,8] Hence, outside of cases clearly illustrated to be paraneoplastic, this article only includes cases in which the malignancy and the paraneoplastic manifestations are diagnosed within 12 months of each other.

Funding sources: none.

Conflicts of interest: none.

[a] Division of Rheumatology, Washington University School of Medicine, 660 South Euclid Avenue, St Louis, MO 63110, USA

[b] Department of Medicine, Washington University School of Medicine, 660 South Euclid Avenue, St Louis, MO 63110, USA

* Corresponding author.

E-mail address: prangana@dom.wustl.edu

Rheum Dis Clin N Am 37 (2011) 593–606

doi:10.1016/j.rdc.2011.09.002

0889-857X/11/$ – see front matter © 2011 Elsevier Inc. All rights reserved.

rheumatic.theclinics.com

Another complicating factor is that most vasculitides, vasculopathies, and hypercoagulable states are thought to be triggered by a particular event, which may include malignancy, in a genetically susceptible host. This may account for the various types of vascular syndromes associated with various malignancies rather than one type of syndrome being associated with a particular neoplasm. Malignancy could serve as a trigger and, once triggered, vasculitis could run a course independent of the malignancy.[9] In this article, only case reports of concordant disease courses will be included (**Box 1**).

PATHOPHYSIOLOGY

The exact pathophysiology of paraneoplastic vascular syndromes is unknown. This article describes pathophysiologic mechanisms as they pertain to each vascular syndrome. In general, proposed mechanisms involve an increased cellular turnover leading to generation of autoantibodies that cannot be appropriately cleared. Whereas this accounts for the increased incidence of autoantibodies found in patients with malignancies, it fails to explain the lack of immune complexes in many paraneoplastic vasculitides.[10] Release of tumor angiogenic factors and/or cytokines, which in turn cause endothelial damage and increased vascular permeability, inflammation, and fibrosis, has been postulated as another potential mechanism.[9,11,12]

Box 1
Neoplastic and paraneoplastic vascular syndromes

Vasculitis

Immune complex–mediated

    Leukocytoclastic vasculitis (Palpable purpura, UV, EED)

    Henoch-Schönlein purpura

    Cryoglobulinemia

ANCA-associated

    Granulomatosis with polyangiitis

    Microscopic polyangiitis

    Churg-Strauss

Other

    Primary angiitis of central nervous system

    Giant cell arteritis

    Polyarteritis nodosa

Vasculopathy

Cutaneous lymphocytic vasculopathy

Raynaud's phenomenon

Erythromelalgia

Hypercoagulability

Thromboembolism

Antiphospholipid antibodies

Abbreviations: ANCA, antineutrophil cytoplasmic antibody; EED, erythema elevatum diutinum; UV, urticarial vasculitis.

Outside of rare associations of particular paraneoplastic vascular syndromes with a specific malignancy (ie, polyarteritis nodosa with hairy cell leukemia), most paraneoplastic vasculitides and vasculopathies are not associated with particular types of malignancy.[11] Although no data currently exist in the literature on this aspect, it would be interesting to determine if patients with a paraneoplastic vasculitis that goes into remission with treatment of the underlying malignancy develop the same type of vasculitis when diagnosed with a new primary malignancy.

VASCULITIDES

Paraneoplastic vasculitides are estimated to represent 2% to 5% of all vasculitides.[1,9,10] Although it is difficult to know whether all were paraneoplastic, vasculitis frequency in cancer patients was estimated at 1 in 1800 for hematologic malignancies and 1 in 80,800 for solid tumors.[13] Like nonneoplastic vasculitides, they are classified by size of vessels involved and presumed pathogenic mechanisms. This article describes three major categories: immune complex–mediated, antineutrophil cytoplasmic antibody (ANCA)-mediated, and other vasculitides that do not fall into the first two categories.

Immune Complex–Mediated Vasculitis

The three well-characterized forms of immune complex–mediated paraneoplastic vasculitis are leukocytoclastic vasculitis (LCV), cryoglobulinemic vasculitis, and Henoch-Schönlein purpura (HSP).

LCV accounts for 50% to 60% of paraneoplastic vasculitis[9,14,15] and is the most frequently seen paraneoplastic vasculitis in both hematologic and solid malignancies. LCV is diagnosed on skin biopsy and it histologically demonstrates neutrophilic inflammation of vessel walls with endothelial swelling and fibrinoid necrosis in postcapillary venules. LCV occurs more frequently in hematologic malignancies and, when present in plasma cell dyscrasias, tends to be due to cryoglobulinemia.[16] There has been no consistent association of LCV with a particular solid tumor. Cases have been reported with lung, prostate, breast, endometrial, ovarian, colon, renal, and head and neck cancers.[10]

Paraneoplastic LCV usually presents as palpable purpura but rare cases of erythema elevatum diutinum (EED) and urticarial vasculitis (UV) have been reported. EED presents as violaceous plaques or nodules found predominantly over the extensor surfaces of hands and elbows,[17] whereas UV (**Fig. 1**) is characterized by erythematous wheals that last for greater than 24 hours. Paraneoplastic EED has

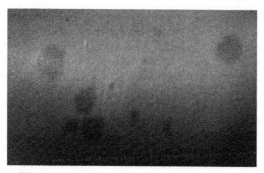

Fig. 1. Urticarial vasculitis.

been reported with breast cancer, B-cell lymphoma, hairy cell leukemia, and lymphoepithelioma-like carcinoma.[17,18] On literature review, only six case reports of paraneoplastic urticarial vasculitis were found: two with Hodgkin's lymphoma,[19] one with non–Hodgkin's lymphoma,[20] two with metastatic colon cancer,[21] and one with malignant teratoma of the testes.[22] Although paraneoplastic cases of EED and UV are rare, numerous cases of medication-induced EED and UV have been reported.[18] Hence, an atypical LCV presentation such as EED and UV would make medication-induced vasculitis more likely than a paraneoplastic process.

Cryoglobulins are cold-precipitated immunoglobulins associated with hepatitis C and HIV infections, lymphoproliferative diseases, and other chronic inflammatory conditions. Neoplastic cryoglobulinemia, accounting for 15% of all cryoglobulinemia, rarely causes vasculitis.[23] Neoplastic cryoglobulinemia is usually monoclonal (type I) and due to lymphoproliferative disorders such as Waldenström's macroglobulinemia, multiple myeloma, non–Hodgkin's lymphoma, and chronic lymphocytic leukemia. Type I cryoglobulins do not have rheumatoid factor activity and, hence, do not easily activate the classical complement pathway. However, a few cases of paraneoplastic cryoglobulinemic vasculitis manifesting only with cutaneous involvement[16,24,25] and one case of type I cryoglobulinemic glomerulonephritis have been described.[24] Most patients with type I cryoglobulins are asymptomatic until concentrations of cryoglobulins reach levels high enough to cause hyperviscosity.[26] Manifestations of hyperviscosity include acrocyanosis, digital gangrene,[27] and strokes.

HSP is an immune complex–mediated small vessel vasculitis defined by IgA deposition in blood vessel walls. Almost all adult patients have palpable purpura and arthralgias, whereas 30% have renal involvement and 50% have gastrointestinal involvement.[28] Paraneoplastic HSP accounts for 15% of paraneoplastic vasculitis[14,15] and occurs more commonly with carcinomas of the lung, urogenital, and gastrointestinal tracts.[29] Zurada and colleagues[30] looked at 31 reported cases of paraneoplastic HSP and noted two key patient characteristics: male gender (95%) and older age (mean age of 68 years with a range of 46–86). When compared with non–malignancy-associated HSP, patients with paraneoplastic HSP tended to have more renal involvement (87%). Mitsui and colleagues[31] retrospectively examined 23 cases of malignancy-associated and 80 cases of non–malignancy-associated HSP during a 20-year period and also found older age (67.2 years vs 41.3 years) to be a risk factor for paraneoplastic HSP but not male gender. Another study comparing 19 HSP patients with known malignancies to 158 HSP patients without a known malignancy concluded that male gender (90% vs 65%) and age greater than 40, combined with a lack of clear infectious or medication triggers, were risk factors for paraneoplastic HSP.[32]

ANCA-Associated Vasculitis

ANCA-associated vasculitides, as a class, is the most common systemic small vessel vasculitis. This class is further divided into granulomatosis with polyangiitis (GPA, formerly known as Wegener's granulomatosis), Churg-Strauss syndrome, and microscopic polyangiitis (MPA) based on clinical manifestations and whether ANCA is perinuclear or cytoplasmic in pattern and whether it binds to myeloperoxidase or proteinase 3.

Although many reports of ANCA-associated vasculitis with a concurrent malignancy exist, paraneoplastic ANCA-associated vasculitides account for less than 5% of paraneoplastic vasculitis, although a positive ANCA can frequently be seen in the setting of malignancy.[9] During an 18.5 year period, Hutson and Hoffman[14] reported one case of GPA, which did not run a concordant course with the patient's malignancy. Solans-Laque and colleagues[15] found no patients with paraneoplastic ANCA-associated vasculitis among 15 patients with paraneoplastic vasculitis during a 15-year period. Tatsis and colleagues[4] reported 14 patients diagnosed with GPA and a concurrent malignancy, but only 4 of the 14 patients had a paraneoplastic manifestation of GPA. Three of the four patients had renal cell carcinomas. One case of paraneoplastic MPA presenting with fevers, mononeuritis multiplex, and glomerulonephritis associated with gastroduodenal carcinoma has been reported.[33] Based on these reports and a retrospective review of 200 patients with MPA or GPA,[34] one can discern that, although paraneoplastic ANCA-associated vasculitis is rare, concurrent diagnoses with independent courses are common. In this study, the largest cohort examined to date, when compared with age-matched groups, the relative risk of having a malignancy at the time of vasculitis diagnosis was 6.02 (95% confidence interval 3.72–9.74).[34]

One case of systemic Churg-Strauss vasculitis associated with recurrence of malignant melanoma has been reported.[35] There are a few case reports of a cutaneous form of Churg-Strauss vasculitis associated with lymphoproliferative disorders.[36–38] These cases are characterized by pruritic nodules on the upper limbs with histology showing dermal eosinophilic collagen necrosis with cellular debris, surrounded by a granulomatous infiltrate of eosinophils and neutrophils.[38]

Other Vasculitis

Primary angiitis of the central nervous system (PACNS) is a rare multifocal, segmental vasculitis affecting the small leptomeningeal and intracerebral arteries. A brain biopsy with surrounding leptomeninges demonstrating vasculitis is the gold standard for diagnosis[39] but, often not obtained owing to its invasive nature. MRI is the most sensitive imaging modality[40] and has a positive predictive value of 43% to 72%, whereas that of cerebral angiography is 37% to 50%. If incidence is based only on cases with confirmed biopsies, paraneoplastic PACNS is rare. Although there are case reports of primary PACNS associated with breast cancer[41] and non–Hodgkin's lymphoma, the strongest association seems to be with Hodgkin's lymphoma because 13 cases have been reported.[42] Symptoms include headaches, seizures, and altered mental status from varied clinical presentations such as encephalopathy, hemorrhage, and infarcts. Unlike other paraneoplastic vasculitides, due to the poor prognosis often associated with paraneoplastic PACNS,[43] the current recommendation is not only to treat the underlying malignancy but to also treat the vasculitis early with corticosteroids and other immunosuppressants.

Giant cell arteritis (GCA) is a large vessel vasculitis predominantly affecting branches of the aorta, especially the extracranial arteries. Many case reports of a synchronous diagnosis of GCA and various malignancies exist,[9,14,15,44–46] but only five cases clearly ran a concordant course with an associated malignancy. The five cases included two cases of lung cancer and one each of cholangiocarcinoma, prostate cancer, and colorectal carcinoma. As a result, some have argued that patients with newly diagnosed GCA have an increased risk of malignancy,[47] but a large prospective case-control study demonstrated no increased risk.[48]

Polyarteritis nodosa (PAN) is a vasculitis affecting small and medium-sized vessels of the peripheral nervous, gastrointestinal, and renal systems. Clinical presentations in paraneoplastic PAN are similar to classical PAN. Paraneoplastic PAN accounts for 15% of all paraneoplastic vasculitides[1,14,15] and, although higher percentages have been cited (around 30%), the cases described in these reports are not clearly demonstrated to be paraneoplastic.[9,49] Paraneoplastic PAN has been frequently described in association with various solid tumors, including bladder,[50] colorectal,[51] gastric,[51] lung,[52] liver,[53] and hypopharyngeal[54] tumors and with hematologic diseases such as myelodysplastic syndrome,[55] hairy cell leukemia[56,57] and chronic myelomonocytic leukemia.[55,58,59]

Of numerous malignancy associations, hairy cell leukemia is the most strongly associated with paraneoplastic PAN. Hairy cell leukemia is a relatively rare leukemia, accounting for only 2% of leukemias.[60] First described by Hughes and colleagues in 1979,[57] the association of hairy cell leukemia and paraneoplastic PAN has been validated by numerous case reports,[60–65] with more than 50 reported cases in literature. Proposed mechanisms for this association include cross-reactivity of antibodies against hairy cell leukemic cell surface antigens and those on vascular endothelial cells.[56,60]

VASCULOPATHY

Neoplastic and paraneoplastic vasculopathy are less frequent than paraneoplastic vasculitides. Much like LCV, cutaneous lymphocytic vasculopathy (CLV) can present as palpable purpura or a maculopapular or papular rash. However, unlike LCV, pruritus is a common symptom. Like LCV, diagnosis is made by biopsy. Histologically, a lymphoplasmacytic perivascular infiltration of the small vessels without significant vessel wall destruction is seen (hence, more of a vasculopathy than a vasculitis). CLV can have various causes, with medications being the number-one offender. Paraneoplastic CLV however, has only been reported in association with lymphoproliferative disorders. One case series reported an incidence of 9.5% among the 116 patients with lymphoproliferative disorders seen at one medical center.[66] Most reported cases were associated with non–Hodgkin's lymphoma or chronic lymphocytic leukemia,[66–68] but CLV has been reported in acute myeloid[69] and lymphoblastic leukemia.[70]

Raynaud's syndrome phenomenon is a vasculopathy characterized by vasospasm of digital arteries resulting in episodic ischemia triggered by cold and emotional stress. The episodic ischemia is characterized by a three-phasic color change of digital tips (pallor, cyanosis, and hyperemia). Unlike CLV, paraneoplastic Raynaud's is not associated with lymphoproliferative disorders but seems to be associated with metastatic solid tumors such as breast,[71] ovarian,[72] lung,[73] head and neck,[74] hepatocellular,[75] and colorectal[76] carcinomas.

Raynaud's as a neoplastic phenomenon was first reported in 1884 in a middle-aged female with breast cancer metastatic to her cervical sympathetic trunk,[77] leading to overstimulation of the sympathetic trunk, much like what is seen with connective tissues diseases. However, subsequent reported cases were deemed paraneoplastic,[72,78] rather than neoplastic, in nature. Determining whether Raynaud's is paraneoplastic or even neoplastic in nature is clouded by the prevalence of idiopathic[78] and chemotherapy-induced Raynaud's,[79–81] leaving some to suggest that Raynaud's does not exist as a paraneoplastic phenomenon. Allen and colleagues[71] compared the characteristics of paraneoplastic Raynaud's with that secondary to chemotherapy and connective tissue diseases and found that paraneoplastic Raynaud's tended to occur in older patients (>50 years), was evenly distributed among men and women, was asymmetric, and progressed much more rapidly to ischemic ulcers and necrosis than the other secondary Raynaud's. Failure of traditional therapies, such as vasodilators and sympathetectomy, may be other clues pointing to paraneoplastic Raynaud's.[67,74,82]

Erythromelalgia (sometimes called erythromalgia) is a rare vasculopathy characterized by intense burning pain, warmth, and erythema precipitated by heat and relieved by elevation and cooling (**Fig. 2**).[83] Erythromelalgia is divided into primary and secondary types, likely involving two distinct pathophysiologic mechanisms. Both primary and secondary erythromelalgia have similar clinical manifestations, but primary erythromelalgia does not respond as well to aspirin therapy. Primary erythromelalgia is considered an autonomic process rather than a vascular phenomenon. The

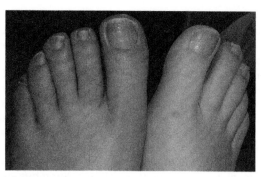

Fig. 2. Erythromelalgia due to thrombocytosis.

few biopsies of primary erythromelalgia suggest no microvascular changes but, instead, suggest decreased autonomic innervation of arteries and sweat glands supplying involved cutaneous areas.[84] Such histopathologic changes suggest that low sympathetic tone leading to impaired vasomotor regulation may be the disease mechanism in primary erythromelalgia.[85]

Secondary erythromelalgia tends to be more asymmetric.[86] There are numerous known causes of secondary erythromelalgia, including, but not limited to, medications, connective tissue diseases, multiple sclerosis, hypertension, and diabetes mellitus. However, one study found that myeloproliferative disorders represent 20% of causes of secondary erythromelalgia.[85] Most cases are reported with polycythemia vera (59%) and essential thrombocythemia (38%). From 50 patients with thrombocytosis related to either polycythemia vera or essential thrombocythemia, Michiels and colleagues[87] found 60% had erythromelalgia. When due to myeloproliferative disorders, if left untreated, secondary erythromelalgia progresses to acrocyanosis and necrosis.[88] The thrombocytosis seen in polycythemia vera and other myeloproliferative disorders may be the mechanism that drives erythromelalgia. Skin biopsies of involved areas show arteriolar thrombosis,[86] whereas platelet hyperaggregability[89] has been described in patients with essential thrombocythemia and erythromelalgia. As a result, pathogenesis is presumed to involve abnormal aggregation of platelets with initially reversible plugging of arterioles.[87]

Although the association between erythromelalgia and myeloproliferative disorders is strong, they likely share a common pathogenic mechanism instead of erythromelalgia being a paraneoplastic syndrome. Only 10% of patients are diagnosed concurrently with erythromelalgia and a myeloproliferative disorder. Erythromelalgia is diagnosed months or even decades ahead of polycythemia vera or essential thrombocythemia.[90] When associated with polycythemia, phlebotomy alleviated symptoms in only a few patients. In thrombocytosis, relapses of erythromelalgia are often seen when platelet counts are greater than $550 \times 10^9/L$, but relapses are not prevented by keeping the platelet count lower.[85] The only treatment consistently effective for both acute episodes and secondary prophylaxis has been aspirin therapy. Aspirin is so unequivocally helpful that some have suggested that response to aspirin therapy be included in the diagnostic criteria for secondary erythromelalgia.[88,90]

HYPERCOAGULABILITY

Epidemiologic studies have identified malignancy as an important risk factor for venous thromboembolism[91] with a reported increased risk of fourfold to sixfold compared with the general population.[92] About 5% of patients with one unprovoked venous thrombus are found to have an occult malignancy. Recurrent venous thromboembolism is four times more likely to be associated with an occult malignancy compared with a single episode of venous thromboembolism.[93]

The pathogenesis of malignancy-related hypercoagulable states is complex but several key players have been identified. Tissue factor expression, a known trigger of the extrinsic coagulation pathway, is normally tightly controlled and is kept to a minimum in vascular cells so that coagulation does not spontaneously occur. However, various solid tumor cell lines demonstrate increased expression of tissue factor[94] to increase secretion of vascular endothelial growth factor,[95,96] a proangiogenic factor, which aids in tumor survival. The increased tissue factor expression increases the risk for thrombus formation without vascular injury.

Another key player is cancer procoagulant, a cysteine protease expressed by various tumor cell lines, including leukemic cells.[97] Cancer procoagulant is able to activate factor X even in the absence of factor VIIa and is thought to contribute much to the heightened coagulopathic state of acute promyelocytic leukemia.[98]

Malignancy-related arterial clots have been reported but are rare when compared with venous thromboembolism. Most cases are related to direct tumor invasion of arteries,[99–101] vasculitis,[102] hyperviscosity, disseminated intravascular coagulation,[103,104] and marantic endocarditis.[105–108] Disseminated intravascular coagulation has been reported to occur in 6.8% of patients with solid organ tumors, most frequently in association with adenocarcinomas.[104]

Antiphospholipid antibodies (aPLs) are known to increase both arterial and venous thrombotic risks. A higher incidence of aPLs was observed in patients with both hematologic disorders,[109] such as myelodysplastic syndrome, lymphoma, and various types of leukemias, as well as solid tumors, such as breast, lung, colon, gastric, thyroid carcinomas.[110] Both Zuckerman and colleagues[110] and Pusterla and colleagues[109] reported an increased incidence of thrombosis in patients with aPLs than in cancer-matched controls. Yet, follow-up of many patients with lymphoproliferative disorders with high titers of aPLs demonstrate that a significant group of patients with aPLs and malignancy do not clinically manifest a thrombus.[111,112] Possibly, as in normal individuals, the presence of aPLs increases the risks of both arterial and venous thrombosis[113] but is not pathogenic in everyone. It is unclear whether patients with positive aPLs would benefit from primary prophylaxis with aspirin or warfarin, given the increased risk of thrombocytopenia and coagulopathies associated with chemotherapy in these same patients.

SUMMARY

It is essential to be aware of both neoplastic and paraneoplastic vasculitides, vasculopathy, and hypercoagulability, considering the importance of an accurate diagnosis and timely treatment of the underlying malignancy. Characteristics such as the type of vasculitis, age, gender, atypical presentation, and lack of response to common therapies should prompt investigation for an occult malignancy, whereas vasculitis such as GPA require due malignancy vigilance given a significantly increased risk of malignancy at the time of diagnosis and in the following years. Vasculopathies are rarer than vasculitides, but are associated with specific malignancies and, in the context of such malignancies, should be kept in mind. Hypercoagulability is a well-documented neoplastic phenomenon with an increased risk of thrombosis in the setting of positive aPLs. Most neoplastic and paraneoplastic vascular syndromes require no specific treatment outside of treatment of the underlying malignancy. The two key exceptions are PACNS, because of its poor prognosis, and erythromelalgia, in which aspirin is an effective agent.

REFERENCES

1. Sanchez-Guerrero J, Gutierrez-Urena S, Vidaller A, et al. Vasculitis as a paraneoplastic syndrome. Report of 11 cases and review of the literature. J Rheumatol 1990;17(11):1458–62.
2. Friedman SA, Bienenstock H, Richter IH. Malignancy and arteriopathy. A report of two cases. Angiology 1969;20(3):136–43.
3. Finazzi G. The Italian registry of antiphospholipid antibodies. Haematologica 1997;82(1):101–5.
4. Tatsis E, Reinhold-Keller E, Steindorf K, et al. Wegener's granulomatosis associated with renal cell carcinoma. Arthritis Rheum 1999;42(4):751–6.
5. Radis CD, Kahl LE, Baker GL, et al. Effects of cyclophosphamide on the development of malignancy and on long-term survival of patients with rheumatoid arthritis. A 20-year followup study. Arthritis Rheum 1995;38(8):1120–7.
6. Kempen JH, Gangaputra S, Daniel E, et al. Long-term risk of malignancy among patients treated with immunosuppressive agents for ocular inflammation: a critical assessment of the evidence. Am J Ophthalmol 2008;146(6). 802–12.e801.
7. Gnanaraj J, Saif MW. Hypersensitivity vasculitis associated with leuprolide (Lupron). Cutan Ocul Toxicol 2010;29(3):224–7.
8. ten Holder SM, Joy MS, Falk RJ. Cutaneous and systemic manifestations of drug-induced vasculitis. Ann Pharmacother 2002;36(1):130–47.
9. Fain O, Hamidou M, Cacoub P, et al. Vasculitides associated with malignancies: analysis of sixty patients. Arthritis Rheum 2007;57(8):1473–80.
10. Garcia-Porrua C, Gonzalez-Gay MA. Cutaneous vasculitis as a paraneoplastic syndrome in adults. Arthritis Rheum 1998;41(6):1133–5.
11. Fortin PR. Vasculitides associated with malignancy. Curr Opin Rheumatol 1996; 8(1):30–3.
12. Buggiani G, Krysenka A, Grazzini M, et al. Paraneoplastic vasculitis and paraneoplastic vascular syndromes. Dermatol Ther 2010;23(6):597–605.
13. Greer JM, Longley S, Edwards NL, et al. Vasculitis associated with malignancy. Experience with 13 patients and literature review. Medicine (Baltimore) 1988; 67(4):220–30.
14. Hutson TE, Hoffman GS. Temporal concurrence of vasculitis and cancer: a report of 12 cases. Arthritis Care Res 2000;13(6):417–23.
15. Solans-Laque R, Bosch-Gil JA, Perez-Bocanegra C, et al. Paraneoplastic vasculitis in patients with solid tumors: report of 15 cases. J Rheumatol 2008;35(2): 294–304.
16. Bayer-Garner IB, Smoller BR. Leukocytoclastic (small vessel) vasculitis in multiple myeloma. Clin Exp Dermatol 2003;28(5):521–4.
17. Liu TC, Chen IS, Lin TK, et al. Erythema elevatum diutinum as a paraneoplastic syndrome in a patient with pulmonary lymphoepithelioma-like carcinoma. Lung Cancer 2009;63(1):151–3.
18. Gibson LE, el-Azhary RA. Erythema elevatum diutinum. Clin Dermatol 2000; 18(3):295–9.
19. Strickland DK, Ware RE. Urticarial vasculitis: an autoimmune disorder following therapy for Hodgkin's disease. Med Pediatr Oncol 1995;25(3):208–12.

20. Wilson D, McCluggage WG, Wright GD. Urticarial vasculitis: a paraneoplastic presentation of B-cell non-Hodgkin's lymphoma. Rheumatology (Oxford) 2002; 41(4):476–7.

21. Lewis JE. Urticarial vasculitis occurring in association with visceral malignancy. Acta Derm Venereol 1990;70(4):345–7.

22. Sprossmann A, Muller RP. Urticaria-vasculitis syndrome in metastatic malignant testicular teratoma. Hautarzt 1994;45(12):871–4 [in German].

23. Dammacco F, Sansonno D, Piccoli C, et al. The cryoglobulins: an overview. Eur J Clin Invest 2001;31(7):628–38.

24. Kim YL, Gong SJ, Hwang YH, et al. Waldenstrom macroglobulinemia with CD5+ expression presented as cryoglobulinemic glomerulonephropathy: a case report. J Korean Med Sci 2011;26(6):824–8.

25. Cem Ar M, Soysal T, Hatemi G, et al. Successful management of cryoglobulinemia-induced leukocytoclastic vasculitis with thalidomide in a patient with multiple myeloma. Ann Hematol 2005;84(9):609–13.

26. Tedeschi A, Barate C, Minola E, et al. Cryoglobulinemia. Blood Rev 2007;21(4): 183–200.

27. Vacula I, Ambrozy E, Makovnik M, et al. Cryoglobulinemia manifested by gangraene of almost all fingers and toes. Int Angiol 2010;29(6):560–4.

28. Pillebout E, Thervet E, Hill G, et al. Henoch-Schonlein Purpura in adults: outcome and prognostic factors. J Am Soc Nephrol 2002;13(5):1271–8.

29. Mifune D, Watanabe S, Kondo R, et al. Henoch Schonlein purpura associated with pulmonary adenocarcinoma. J Med Case Reports 2011;5(1):226.

30. Zurada JM, Ward KM, Grossman ME. Henoch-Schonlein purpura associated with malignancy in adults. J Am Acad Dermatol 2006;55(Suppl 5): S65–70.

31. Mitsui H, Shibagaki N, Kawamura T, et al. A clinical study of Henoch-Schonlein Purpura associated with malignancy. J Eur Acad Dermatol Venereol 2009;23(4): 394–401.

32. Pertuiset E, Liote F, Launay-Russ E, et al. Adult Henoch-Schonlein purpura associated with malignancy. Semin Arthritis Rheum 2000;29(6):360–7.

33. Abe H, Momose S, Takeuchi T. Microscopic polyangitis complicating double carcinoma of the stomach and duodenum: improvement after the resection of these carcinomas. Rheumatol Int 2011;31(1):105–8.

34. Pankhurst T, Savage CO, Gordon C, et al. Malignancy is increased in ANCA-associated vasculitis. Rheumatology (Oxford) 2004;43(12):1532–5.

35. Cupps TR, Fauci AS. Neoplasm and systemic vasculitis: a case report. Arthritis Rheum 1982;25(4):475–6.

36. Finan MC, Winkelmann RK. The cutaneous extravascular necrotizing granuloma (Churg-Strauss granuloma) and systemic disease: a review of 27 cases. Medicine (Baltimore) 1983;62(3):142–58.

37. Finan MC, Winkelmann RK. Cutaneous extravascular necrotizing granuloma and lymphocytic lymphoma. Arch Dermatol 1983;119(5):419–22.

38. Calonje JE, Greaves MW. Cutaneous extravascular necrotizing granuloma (Churg-Strauss) as a paraneoplastic manifestation of non-Hodgkin's B-cell lymphoma. J R Soc Med 1993;86(9):549–50.

39. Calabrese LH, Furlan AJ, Gragg LA, et al. Primary angiitis of the central nervous system: diagnostic criteria and clinical approach. Cleve Clin J Med 1992;59(3): 293–306.

40. Chu CT, Gray L, Goldstein LB, et al. Diagnosis of intracranial vasculitis: a multi-disciplinary approach. J Neuropathol Exp Neurol 1998;57(1):30–8.

41. Taccone FS, Salmon I, Marechal R, et al. Paraneoplastic vasculitis of central nervous system presenting as recurrent cryptogenic stroke. Int J Clin Oncol 2007;12(2):155–9.

42. Rosen CL, DePalma L, Morita A. Primary angiitis of the central nervous system as a first presentation in Hodgkin's disease: a case report and review of the literature. Neurosurgery 2000;46(6):1504–8 [discussion: 1508–10].

43. Woolfenden AR, Tong DC, Marks MP, et al. Angiographically defined primary angiitis of the CNS: is it really benign? Neurology 1998;51(1):183–8.

44. Kurzrock R, Cohen PR, Markowitz A. Clinical manifestations of vasculitis in patients with solid tumors. A case report and review of the literature. Arch Intern Med 1994;154(3):334–40.

45. Hauser WA, Ferguson RH, Holley KE, et al. Temporal arteritis in Rochester, Minnesota, 1951 to 1967. Mayo Clin Proc 1971;46(9):597–602.

46. Liozon E, Loustaud V, Fauchais AL, et al. Concurrent temporal (giant cell) arteritis and malignancy: report of 20 patients with review of the literature. J Rheumatol 2006;33(8):1606–14.

47. von Knorring J, Somer T. Malignancy in association with polymyalgia rheumatica and temporal arteritis. Scand J Rheumatol 1974;3(3):129–35.

48. Myklebust G, Wilsgaard T, Jacobsen BK, et al. No increased frequency of malignant neoplasms in polymyalgia rheumatica and temporal arteritis. A prospective longitudinal study of 398 cases and matched population controls. J Rheumatol 2002;29(10):2143–7.

49. Fain O, Guillevin L, Kaplan G, et al. Vasculitis and neoplasms. 14 cases. Ann Med Interne (Paris) 1991;142(7):486–504 [in French].

50. Hayem G, Gomez MJ, Grossin M, et al. Systemic vasculitis and epithelioma. A report of three cases with a literature review. Rev Rhum Engl Ed 1997;64(12):816–24.

51. Paajanen H, Heikkinen M, Tarvainen R, et al. Anaplastic colon carcinoma associated with necrotizing vasculitis. J Clin Gastroenterol 1995;21(2):168–9.

52. Beji M, Khedher I, Ayadi N, et al. Periarteritis nodosa associated with lung cancer. A new observation. Tunis Med 1999;77(11):585–8 [in French].

53. Minakuchi K, Fujimoto K, Takada K, et al. Hepatocellular carcinoma associated with polyarteritis nodosa with symptoms appearing after intra-arterial chemotherapy. Br J Radiol 1991;64(759):272–5.

54. Okada M, Suzuki K, Hidaka T, et al. Polyarteritis associated with hypopharyngeal carcinoma. Intern Med 2002;41(10):892–5.

55. Saif MW, Hopkins JL, Gore SD. Autoimmune phenomena in patients with myelodysplastic syndromes and chronic myelomonocytic leukemia. Leuk Lymphoma 2002;43(11):2083–92.

56. Vankalakunti M, Joshi K, Jain S, et al. Polyarteritis nodosa in hairy cell leukaemia: an autopsy report. J Clin Pathol 2007;60(10):1181–2.

57. Hughes GR, Elkon KB, Spiller R, et al. Polyarteritis nodosa and hairy-cell leukaemia. Lancet 1979;1(8117):678.

58. Hamidou MA, Boumalassa A, Larroche C, et al. Systemic medium-sized vessel vasculitis associated with chronic myelomonocytic leukemia. Semin Arthritis Rheum 2001;31(2):119–26.

59. Paydas S, Zorludemir S, Sahin B. Vasculitis and leukemia. Leuk Lymphoma 2000;40(1–2):105–12.

60. Hasler P, Kistler H, Gerber H. Vasculitides in hairy cell leukemia. Semin Arthritis Rheum 1995;25(2):134–42.

61. Carpenter MT, West SG. Polyarteritis nodosa in hairy cell leukemia: treatment with interferon-alpha. J Rheumatol 1994;21(6):1150–2.

62. Komadina KH, Houk RW. Polyarteritis nodosa presenting as recurrent pneumonia following splenectomy for hairy-cell leukemia. Semin Arthritis Rheum 1989;18(4):252–7.

63. Thorwarth WT Jr, Jaques PF, Orringer EP. Polyarteritis nodosa in hairy cell leukemia. J Can Assoc Radiol 1983;34(2):151–2.

64. Le Pogamp P, Ghandour C, Le Prise PY. Hairy Cell leukemia and polyarteritis nodosa. J Rheumatol 1982;9(3):441–2.

65. Goedert JJ, Neefe JR, Smith FS, et al. Polyarteritis nodosa, hairy cell leukemia and splenosis. Am J Med 1981;71(2):323–6.

66. Pavlidis NA, Klouvas G, Tsokos M, et al. Cutaneous lymphocytic vasculopathy in lymphoproliferative disorders–a paraneoplastic lymphocytic vasculitis of the skin. Leuk Lymphoma 1995;16(5–6):477–82.

67. Cabuk M, Inanir I, Turkdogan P, et al. Cyclic lymphocytic vasculitis associated with chronic lymphocytic leukemia. Leuk Lymphoma 2004;45(4):811–3.

68. Robak E, Robak T. Skin lesions in chronic lymphocytic leukemia. Leuk Lymphoma 2007;48(5):855–65.

69. Farrell AM, Gooptu C, Woodrow D, et al. Cutaneous lymphocytic vasculitis in acute myeloid leukaemia. Br J Dermatol 1996;135(3):471–4.

70. Jaing TH, Hsueh C, Chiu CH, et al. Cutaneous lymphocytic vasculitis as the presenting feature of acute lymphoblastic leukemia. J Pediatr Hematol Oncol 2002; 24(7):555–7.

71. Allen D, Robinson D, Mittoo S. Paraneoplastic Raynaud's phenomenon in a breast cancer survivor. Rheumatol Int 2010;30(6):789–92.

72. Kohli M, Bennett RM. Raynaud's phenomenon as a presenting sign of ovarian adenocarcinoma. J Rheumatol 1995;22(7):1393–4.

73. Kopterides P, Tsavaris N, Tzioufas A, et al. Digital gangrene and Raynaud's phenomenon as complications of lung adenocarcinoma. Lancet Oncol 2004; 5(9):549.

74. Wright JR, Gudelis S. Digital necrosis associated with squamous cell carcinoma of the tonsil. Head Neck 2002;24(11):1019–21.

75. Sahan C, Ucer T, Aksakal E. A case of hepatocellular carcinoma who admitted with Raynaud's phenomenon. Rheumatol Int 2006;27(1):87–9.

76. Paw P, Dharan SM, Sackier JM. Digital ischemia and occult malignancy. Int J Colorectal Dis 1996;11(4):196–7.

77. O'Connor B. Symmetrical gangrene. Br Med J 1884;1(1210):460.

78. Wigley FM, Flavahan NA. Raynaud's phenomenon. Rheum Dis Clin North Am 1996;22(4):765–81.

79. De Angelis R, Silveri F, Bugatti L, et al. Raynaud's phenomenon after combined adjuvant chemotherapy for breast cancer. Chemotherapy 2003;49(5):267–8.

80. Papamichael D, Amft N, Slevin ML, et al. 5-Fluorouracil-induced Raynaud's phenomenon. Eur J Cancer 1998;34(12):1983.

81. Toumbis-Ioannou E, Cohen PR. Chemotherapy-induced Raynaud's phenomenon. Cleve Clin J Med 1994;61(3):195–9.

82. Naschitz JE, Rosner I, Rozenbaum M, et al. Rheumatic syndromes: clues to occult neoplasia. Semin Arthritis Rheum 1999;29(1):43–55.

83. Mitchell SW. On a rare vasomotor neurosis of the extremities, and on the maladies with which it may be confounded. Am J Med Sci 1878;76:17–36.

84. Uno H, Parker F. Autonomic innervation of the skin in primary erythermalgia. Arch Dermatol 1983;119(1):65–71.

85. Kurzrock R, Cohen PR. Erythromelalgia and myeloproliferative disorders. Arch Intern Med 1989;149(1):105–9.
86. Michiels JJ, Abels J, Steketee J, et al. Erythromelalgia caused by platelet-mediated arteriolar inflammation and thrombosis in thrombocythemia. Ann Intern Med 1985;102(4):466–71.
87. Michiels JJ, ten Kate FJ. Erythromelalgia in thrombocythemia of various myeloproliferative disorders. Am J Hematol 1992;39(2):131–6.
88. Michiels JJ, Berneman Z, Schroyens W, et al. Aspirin-responsive painful red, blue, black toe, or finger syndrome in polycythemia vera associated with thrombocythemia. Ann Hematol 2003;82(3):153–9.
89. Boneu B, Pris J, Guiraud B, et al. Abnormalities of platelet aggregation during essential thrombocythemia. Effect of aspirin on erythromelalgia. Nouv Presse Med 1972;1(36):2383–8 [in French].
90. Babb RR, Alarcon-Segovia D, Fairbairn JF 2nd. Erythermalgia. Review of 51 Cases. Circulation 1964;29:136–41.
91. Levitan N, Dowlati A, Remick SC, et al. Rates of initial and recurrent thromboembolic disease among patients with malignancy versus those without malignancy. Risk analysis using Medicare claims data. Medicine (Baltimore) 1999;78(5):285–91.
92. Heit JA, Silverstein MD, Mohr DN, et al. Risk factors for deep vein thrombosis and pulmonary embolism: a population-based case-control study. Arch Intern Med 2000;160(6):809–15.
93. Prandoni P, Lensing AW, Buller HR, et al. Deep-vein thrombosis and the incidence of subsequent symptomatic cancer. N Engl J Med 1992;327(16):1128–33.
94. Semeraro N, Colucci M. Tissue factor in health and disease. Thromb Haemost 1997;78(1):759–64.
95. Winter PC. The pathogenesis of venous thromboembolism in cancer: emerging links with tumour biology. Hematol Oncol 2006;24(3):126–33.
96. Nagy JA, Benjamin L, Zeng H, et al. Vascular permeability, vascular hyperpermeability and angiogenesis. Angiogenesis 2008;11(2):109–19.
97. Olas B, Mielicki WP, Wachowicz B, et al. Cancer procoagulant stimulates platelet adhesion. Thromb Res 1999;94(3):199–203.
98. Gordon SG, Cross BA. A factor X-activating cysteine protease from malignant tissue. J Clin Invest 1981;67(6):1665–71.
99. Jimenez-Jaimez J, Macias-Ruiz R, Montes-Ramirez JM. Diffuse large B-cell lymphoma presenting as an intracardiac mass. J Am Coll Cardiol 2009;53(9):811.
100. Levi M, Bronkhorst C, Noorduyn LA, et al. Recurrent thrombotic occlusions of arteries and veins caused by intravascular metastatic adenocarcinoma. J Clin Pathol 1994;47(9):858–9.
101. Sibbing D, Barthel P, Abbrederis K, et al. Intracardiac right ventricular metastatic tumor of malignant T-cell lymphoma. Int J Cardiol 2007;117(2):e84–5.
102. Roggerone S, Traverse-Glehen A, Derex L, et al. Recurrent cerebral venous thrombosis revealing paraneoplastic angiitis in Hodgkin's lymphoma. J Neurooncol 2008;89(2):195–8.
103. Voulgaris E, Pentheroudakis G, Vassou A, et al. Disseminated intravascular coagulation (DIC) and non-small cell lung cancer (NSCLC): report of a case and review of the literature. Lung Cancer 2009;64(2):247–9.
104. Sallah S, Wan JY, Nguyen NP, et al. Disseminated intravascular coagulation in solid tumors: clinical and pathologic study. Thromb Haemost 2001;86(3):828–33.

105. Glass JP. The diagnosis and treatment of stroke in a patient with cancer: nonbacterial thrombotic endocarditis (NBTE): a case report and review. Clin Neurol Neurosurg 1993;95(4):315–8.
106. Lal G, Brennan TV, Hambleton J, et al. Coagulopathy, marantic endocarditis, and cerebrovascular accidents as paraneoplastic features in medullary thyroid cancer—case report and review of the literature. Thyroid 2003;13(6):601–5.
107. Marglani O, Al-Herabi A, Odell P. Marantic endocarditis as an unusual paraneoplastic syndrome of head and neck squamous cell carcinoma. J Otolaryngol Head Neck Surg 2009;38(2):E76–7.
108. Warkentin TE, Whitlock RP, Teoh KH. Warfarin-associated multiple digital necrosis complicating heparin-induced thrombocytopenia and Raynaud's phenomenon after aortic valve replacement for adenocarcinoma-associated thrombotic endocarditis. Am J Hematol 2004;75(1):56–62.
109. Pusterla S, Previtali S, Marziali S, et al. Antiphospholipid antibodies in lymphoma: prevalence and clinical significance. Hematol J 2004;5(4):341–6.
110. Zuckerman E, Toubi E, Golan TD, et al. Increased thromboembolic incidence in anti-cardiolipin-positive patients with malignancy. Br J Cancer 1995;72(2): 447–51.
111. Miesbach W, Scharrer I, Asherson RA. High titres of IgM-antiphospholipid antibodies are unrelated to pathogenicity in patients with non-Hodgkin's lymphoma. Clin Rheumatol 2007;26(1):95–7.
112. Genvresse I, Luftner D, Spath-Schwalbe E, et al. Prevalence and clinical significance of anticardiolipin and anti-beta2-glycoprotein-I antibodies in patients with non-Hodgkin's lymphoma. Eur J Haematol 2002;68(2):84–90.
113. Genvresse I, Buttgereit F, Spath-Schwalbe E, et al. Arterial thrombosis associated with anticardiolipin and anti-beta2-glycoprotein-I antibodies in patients with non-Hodgkin's lymphoma: a report of two cases. Eur J Haematol 2000; 65(5):344–7.

Paraneoplastic Myalgias and Myositis

Rohit Aggarwal, MD, MS[a],*, Chester V. Oddis, MD[b]

KEYWORDS

• Cancer • Myositis • Paraneoplastic

The idiopathic inflammatory myopathies (IIMs) are a group of acquired, heterogeneous, connective tissue diseases that mainly affect skeletal muscle. Characteristic clinical and histopathologic features allow their classification into polymyositis (PM), dermatomyositis (DM), and inclusion body myositis (IBM). The association between cancer and IIM has been extensively reported in adults, although the pathogenesis remains elusive. Several epidemiologic studies have confirmed the increased risk of cancer in patients with myositis, particularly in DM patients compared with other myositis subsets. Although cancer-associated myositis (CAM) has a worse prognosis in afflicted patients, its timely recognition is therapeutically important and certainly contributes to morbidity and mortality. In this article, the authors discuss several aspects of CAM including epidemiology, risk factors, autoantibody associations, pathophysiology, and screening.

EPIDEMIOLOGY

Several epidemiologic studies have reported the association between cancer and myositis for nearly 100 years. Since 1916, when the first case reports of malignancies occurring in patients with both DM and PM were described, many studies have substantiated this association and attempted to understand the complex relationship between these 2 entities. Early reports included case–control studies and were limited by a lack of standardized definitions, referral bias, small sample sizes, and other methodological shortcomings. Moreover, amyopathic DM and necrotizing myopathy, 2 more recently described myositis subsets, were not well recognized. In the last decade, large population-based epidemiologic studies from the Scandinavian countries, Australia, and Scotland have confirmed the increased risk of malignancy in

---

[a] Division of Rheumatology and Clinical Immunology, University of Pittsburgh, 3601 5th Avenue, Suite 2B, 243, Pittsburgh, PA 15213, USA
[b] Division of Rheumatology and Clinical Immunology, University of Pittsburgh, 3500 Terrace Street, BST S 705, Pittsburgh, PA 15261, USA
* Corresponding author.
E-mail address: aggarwalr@upmc.edu

Rheum Dis Clin N Am 37 (2011) 607–621
doi:10.1016/j.rdc.2011.09.007
0889-857X/11/$ – see front matter © 2011 Elsevier Inc. All rights reserved.

patients with inflammatory myopathy.[1–4] Most studies estimate a frequency of cancer in adult patients with myositis between 10% and 30%, with DM representing the greatest risk factor.

In 2001, Hill described the temporal link between myositis and malignancy[2] in a pooled analysis of national cancer registry databases using discharge diagnoses from Sweden, Finland, and Denmark. Standardized incidence ratios (SIRs), the observed incidence of malignancy in the myositis cohort compared with the expected rates in the general population, were 3.0 for DM and 1.4 for PM. Specifically 618 DM and 914 PM patients met Bohan and Peter criteria, with a cancer frequency of approximately 30% in DM and 15% in PM patients. Sixty percent of tumors were diagnosed after the diagnosis of myositis, and most cancers were detected within 1 year of patients developing myositis. As seen in earlier observational studies, the most common cancer types were adenocarcinomas, which accounted for 70% of all associated tumors. A major limitation of this study was the lack of biopsy-proven myositis and little ethnic diversity, suggesting that their results are mainly relevant for Caucasians. Another large epidemiologic study using state cancer registry databases and the national death index identified 74 (14%) cancer cases in a population-based retrospective cohort of 537 patients with biopsy-proven IIM.[1] Malignancy was diagnosed concurrently (within 7 days) or after the diagnosis of myositis, and the overall risk for cancer in IIM was overall 2 to 3-fold higher (SIR 2.6), greatest in DM (SIR, 6.2 [confidence interval, CI, 3.9–10.0]) but also increased in PM (SIR, 2.0 [CI, 1.4–2.7]). In a meta-analysis, Zantos analyzed 1078 patients with PM/DM (565/513) from four different studies with a comparable number of controls. One hundred fifty-three myositis patients had cancer within 10 years of diagnosis, with the findings supporting an association of both PM and DM with cancer. An overall combined relative risk of cancer was 4.4 (9.5% CI 3.0, 6.6) and 2.1 (95% CI 1.4, 3.3) in DM and PM, respectively.[5]

In contrast with large studies demonstrating a significant relationship between PM and cancer,[1–6] Antiochos reported no association of cancer with PM.[7] Similarly, Airio also observed a higher relative risk of cancer (SIR 6.5, 95% CI 3.9–10) among patients with DM but not in patients with PM in a population-based study of myositis in Finland.[8]

Association Between Histologic Types of Cancer and Myositis

In DM, all histologic types of cancer have an increased risk, but adenocarcinomas are the most common. In contrast, hematological malignancies have the highest risk in PM, with no increase observed in the risk of squamous cell cancers and adenocarcinomas.[2] Although a wide spectrum of cancer types can be associated with myositis, certain types are more frequent and may help guide the workup for occult malignancy. Most studies show the highest risk of lung, ovarian, cervical, colorectal, gastric, breast, and pancreatic cancer along with lymphomas in DM. In PM, the greatest increased risks were for lymphoma in most studies, and lung and bladder cancers in some studies, and there was no increased risk of ovarian, colorectal, stomach, or pancreatic cancers.[2,4]

Temporal Relationship Between Time of IIM Diagnosis and Cancer Risk

Cancer can be diagnosed before, concurrent with, or after the diagnosis of inflammatory myopathy. The peak incidence of malignancy (PM/DM combined) is highest within the first year of myositis diagnosis (60%–70% cases) and decreases substantially each year thereafter. The overall interval with highest probability for tumor recognition is generally between 2 years preceding and 3 years following the diagnosis of myositis.[9] In most studies, the risk of cancer in DM extends up to 5 years, while the cancer risk in PM appears to be shorter. In Hill's study, the risk of cancer in PM was much lower after the first year of diagnosis, and fell to the expected baseline risk of cancer in the general population within 5 years of diagnosis. In DM, the higher risk of most cancers extended up to 5 years, and in colorectal and pancreatic cancer, the risk extended beyond 5 years. The risk of non-Hodgkin lymphoma in both DM and PM was only increased in the first year.[2] A similar decreasing trend in the risk of malignancy was observed each year after the diagnosis of myositis (PM and DM) by Buchbinder, with SIR of 4.4 (CI 2.7–7.1) in the first year; 3.4 (CI, 2.3–5.1) between 1 and 3 years; 2.2 (CI, 1.3–3.9) between 3 and 5 years; and 1.6 (CI, 1.0 –2.6) beyond 5 years.[1] This risk of cancer in DM reaches the baseline general population risk after 5 years when adjusted for age, gender, and calendar year. Of cancers diagnosed before DM, the risk was increased up to 2 years before diagnosis, whereas in PM there appears to be no increase risk before 1 year before diagnosis in most studies.[2] One meta-analysis noted no increase risk of cancer before the diagnosis of PM.[5]

Relationship of Age, Gender and Ethnicity with CAM

The mean age of CAM approximates 50 to 60 years of age, although the range is wide. The risk of cancer associated with DM appears higher (more than 3-fold in most studies) in patients 45 years and older, as compared with younger patients (2-fold increase for 15–44 years).[4,7,9] In PM, older patients are more at risk in most studies, but Stockton showed the risk was higher in the 15 to 44 age group in PM as compared with patients 45 to 74 years old.[4] Many studies show an increased risk of malignancy with increased age.[6,8,10–12]

The risk of cancer is increased in both men and women, although many but not all studies suggest a slightly higher risk for men. The SIRs for men and women with DM were 3.3 (95% CI 2.5–4.4) and 2.8 (2.2–3.6), respectively. The SIR for PM was 1.4 (95% CI 1.0–1.8) for men and 1.2 (0.9–1.6) for women.[2] There was no difference in the rate of sex-neutral cancers between male or female.[7]

The epidemiology of CAM is very different in some nonwhite ethnicities. Breast, stomach, and nasopharyngeal cancer (NPC) are more common with DM in Korea,[13] while NPC is the most CAM malignancy in Singapore, Hong Kong, southeastern China, and Taiwan.[10,14,15]

Risk of Cancer in Other Myositis Subsets

One population based study found an increased risk for malignancy in IBM (SIR, 2.4 [CI, 1.2–4.9]), myositis associated with connective tissue disease (SIR, 4.6 [CI, 1.2–11.7]), and childhood myositis (SIR, 29.0 [CI, 3.5–105.0]).[1] Others have also noted this malignancy association with juvenile DM (JDM), amyopathic DM (ADM), and IBM,[1,16–20] with further substantiation in ADM.[21] However, these associations need to be confirmed by larger population-based studies.

Survival in CAM

The type and stage of the underlying malignancy and the presence of severe myositis features such as respiratory insufficiency and dysphagia determine the prognosis of CAM. One-year survival and 5-year survival were significantly higher in non-CAM (95% and 92%) as compared with patients with CAM (88% and 66%).[9] Increased mortality was also noted in an earlier study, with death rates of 75% in CAM (both PM and DM) compared with 12.5% in non-CAM (P<.001), and death always resulted from progression of the malignancy.[22] In patients where cancer and DM are simultaneously diagnosed, the disease course is more severe than those where the tumor is diagnosed before myositis.[9]

Controversies Regarding the Relationship Between Cancer and Myositis

Although epidemiologic studies have confirmed the association between cancer and myositis, the question of increased cancer surveillance contributing to this relationship persists. This is doubtful for several reasons:

In DM the increased risk of cancer persists for several years of follow-up.

There is a clustering of cancer cases before the diagnosis of myositis.

Mortality due to cancer is increased in DM, which would not be affected by the fortuitous diagnosis of malignant disease.

An increased risk of malignancy in the time following the diagnosis of DM has been noted even when the initial year of follow-up is excluded.[1,2,4,5]

In contrast, increased surveillance for cancer as well as misclassification of DM as PM could partially contribute to the greater risk in PM. A meta-analysis of case-control and cohort studies of myositis and malignant disease showed no increase in cancer detection before the diagnosis of PM, despite a raised risk after diagnosis.[5] Similarly, only Caucasian patients with DM and not PM from northern New England showed a high risk of developing cancer.[7] However, Buchbinder, who classified myositis histologically and was less likely to have misclassified DM and PM, showed a small but significant increased risk of malignant disease in PM.[1] A slight but increased risk of malignant disease in PM seems likely.

Effects of CAM Treatment on Myositis

Although treatment of the tumor (surgery, chemotherapy, radiotherapy) may lead to remission of the myositis,[9] many patients require long-term immunosuppression to control myositis even with cancer remission. Myositis can recur upon relapse of malignancy even years after initial presentation.

RISK FACTORS FOR CAM

Identifying IIM patients at risk of developing malignancy has clear importance to the managing clinician. Older age, male sex, refractory or recurrent myositis, severe muscle weakness including respiratory muscle weakness and dysphagia, and skin manifestations such as necrosis, periungual erythema, and the V or shawl sign are associated with occult malignancy in patients with myositis.[9,10,23] Treatment-resistant skin changes (eg, ulcerations and necrosis) are observed more commonly in CAM (44% vs 12%, $P<.05$).[9] Necrotizing cutaneous lesions and severe pruritus are predictive factors for CAM,[24,25] and leukocytoclastic vasculitis has been seen in patients with DM and malignancy.[26]

The muscle weakness of CAM is generally rapidly progressive and severe, leading to immobility (39% vs 12%, $P<.05$) and may be distal in location as well (57% vs 6%, $P<.05$). Dysphagia (50% vs 36%), oropharyngeal dysfunction (32% vs 13%), and respiratory muscle involvement (32% vs 16%, $P<.05$) are more frequent in CAM, and respiratory insufficiency due to respiratory muscle involvement can be fatal.[9,27] Joint symptoms (16% vs 51%, $P<.05$), Raynaud syndrome (11% vs 26%, $P<.05$), and fever (0% vs 29%, $P<.05$) were less common in CAM[9] and may be protective.[10,28] In a univariate analysis of 121 patients with DM compared with 29 patients with CAM seen over 13 years, male sex, an older age at presentation, the acute onset of cutaneous or muscular symptoms, periungual erythema, necrotic skin lesions, higher creatine kinase (CK) levels, antinuclear antibody titers, and lower C4 and C3 levels were associated with underlying malignancy in DM patients.[29] In the subsequent multivariate analysis, age over 52, rapid onset of skin or muscle symptoms, cutaneous necrosis, periungual erythema, and low C4 levels were the only factors associated with higher risk of CAM.

The presence of interstitial lung disease (ILD) and antisynthetase autoantibodies seems to be protective for the development of cancer,[9,11] and some report no cases of ILD among patients with cancer in any of the IIM subsets (estimated OR 0.07, 95% CI 0.004–1.18).[7] Earlier studies report similar findings,[10,23] and many investigators note a lower frequency or absence of anti-Jo-1 autoantibody in the sera of CAM patients.[7,9,30,31] However, case reports of malignancy in patients with ILD and anti-Jo-1 antibodies have surfaced,[32–34] so a positive Jo-1 autoantibody and ILD do not preclude a consideration of malignancy in certain clinical settings. Moreover, several cases of ILD in CAM patients noted a fulminant course leading to death from respiratory insufficiency before the malignancy work-up was completed.[35,36]

Although the data indicate that the absence of the more commonly available serologies confers a greater risk of malignancy, autoantibodies are not entirely protective against CAM. A positive antinuclear antibody (ANA) and extractable nuclear antigen were significantly more frequent in idiopathic myositis as compared with CAM.[7,9] Similarly, positive myositis-specific and myositis-associated antibodies (for example anti-PM-Scl, anti-Ro, antisynthetase antibodies) are less frequently associated with CAM.[23]

Despite the severity of myopathic symptoms in CAM, the serum CK and lactate dehydrogenase (LDH) levels were often less elevated,[9] and may be within the normal range.[2,37] However, the reverse has also been reported.[7,29] An interesting association between severe capillary derangement on capillaroscopy and CAM has been found (3 of 6 in CAM vs 3 of 47 in non-CAM patients) (odds ratio [OR] 14.7; 95% CI, 2.0–106.6).[38]

There are no characteristic histopathologic findings in patients with myositis that consistently raise the suspicion of an associated occult malignancy. Nevertheless, necrotizing myopathy with pipestem microvascular changes has been associated with cancer.[39] Muscle biopsy specimens characteristically show evidence of massive necrosis of the muscle fibers with almost complete absence of inflammatory infiltrates, perhaps suggesting involvement of humoral immunologic mechanisms directed against tumor cells.

AUTOANTIBODIES ASSOCIATED WITH CAM

No specific or sensitive clinical or biologic marker for the diagnosis of CAM has been identified. As noted previously, the absence of autoantibodies may predict a higher risk of occult malignancy, whereas the presence of antisynthetase autoantibodies seems to be protective against cancer.[9,10,23] To achieve a higher predictive value for diagnosing CAM, Chinoy and colleagues[11] cross-sectionally determined the antibody profile of Caucasian myositis patients from the United Kingdom, specifically assessing anti-Jo-1, anti-PM-Scl, anti-U1-RNP, anti-U3-RNP, and anti-Ku antibodies. They found a paucity of these autoantibodies in CAM patients quantifying a 6- to 7-fold increased relative cancer risk in individuals lacking this panel of autoantibodies compared with those possessing such antibodies. Finding this panel of autoantibodies negative had a high negative predictive value for CAM, perhaps helpful to managing clinicians until better predictive markers are commercially available. However, other authors have not confirmed these findings, perhaps related to examining fewer cases, which limited the statistical power.[40]

Antl-MI-2 is associated with skin changes and possible occult malignancy in some patients with DM.[41,42] A large study of white patients with myositis found a low prevalence of anti-Mi-2 antibodies in CAM,[43] while a European study suggested that cancer risk was increased, but only in anti-Mi-2 antibody-positive patients possessing the N-terminal fragment of the Mi-2 antigen.[44]

A newly described autoantibody (anti-p155) against a 155-kDa nuclear protein, identified as transcription intermediary factor 1-gamma (TIF1-g), has proven useful for cancer screening in patients with DM. This marker is also found in JDM but is not associated with cancer in this IIM subset as opposed to adults having an increased risk of CAM who possess this autoantibody.[45] A recent study proposed that anti-p155 is involved in the transforming growth factor beta (TGF-β) signaling pathway, which is inactivated in some malignancies, thus linking TIF1-γ to carcinogenesis. The association between adult CAM and anti-p155 has been confirmed in other case series.[11,46–48] Possession of the anti-p155 autoantibody represents a significant risk factor for CAM, and it was found exclusively in DM with a high negative predictive value for CAM. Its role in PM is unclear and requires further investigation. The value of anti-p155 to predict the existence of occult cancer seems to be limited to DM patients, the most highly affected myositis subset for cancer.

In a recent meta-analysis of six published reports, anti-p155 was associated with cancer, with an overall specificity of 70%, sensitivity of 89%, negative predictive value (NPV) of 93%, and a diagnostic odds ratio of 18 (95% CI 8–40).[49] Thus, 70% of myositis patients with anti-p155 will develop cancer, and positive testing leads to an 18-fold higher association with cancer than anti-p155 negative status. Thus, this autoantibody is potentially very helpful in the work-up and follow-up of myositis patients. Moreover, additional studies suggest that ILD and positive antisynthetase autoantibodies or the presence of anti-Mi-2 (subunit Mi-2b), previously reported to be protective or associated with cancer, respectively, were congruent with positive or negative anti-p155 autoantibodies.

Chinoy and colleagues combined the results of the aforementioned autoantibody panel (anti-Jo-1, anti-Ku, anti-PM-Scl, anti-U1-RNP, anti-U3 - RNP) and anti-p155 testing in a cohort of 282 myositis patients to predict CAM.[11] They showed that a negative autoantibody panel alone was highly sensitive (87%) and had high NPV (98%), but low specificity (45%) for CAM. A positive anti-p155 alone was 50% sensitive for the detection of CAM with a 42% positive predictive value (PPV) (ie, 58% false-positive rate). However, the anti-p155 antibody test was 96% specific (most non-CAM patients were negative for this antibody) and demonstrated a high NPV (97% of patients without anti-p155 antibody did not have CAM). Finally, when the autoantibody panel and anti-p155 were negative, there was 94% sensitivity and 99% NPV (indicating that only 1% with a negative autoantibody panel or a negative anti-p155 had CAM). When the DM group was analyzed alone, this combined strategy yielded 100% sensitivity and NPV. However, the specificity and PPV of the combined strategy was low, at 45% and 9%, respectively, indicating these tests are most helpful to rule out malignancies, since positive anti-p155 autoantibody results can be seen in many patients without CAM.

The factors that lead to the development of cancer in some patients with this autoantibody remain unclear and warrants further investigation. It is possible that different epitopes or varying titers of anti-p155 lead to different clinical risk and phenotypes. Moreover, longitudinal measurement of these autoantibodies may provide further information on risk and prognosis of cancer and myositis in patients possessing this marker. Commercial testing of this autoantibody is not yet available.

PATHOGENESIS OF CAM

Several theories have been proposed to explain the association of myositis with cancer[37]:

Paraneoplastic syndromes—bioactive mediators produced by the tumor induce immune reactions against muscle fibers and skin

Causal role of a compromised immune system in the coexistent outbreak of tumor and myositis[8]

Malignant transformation induced by cytotoxic agents used in the treatment of myositis

Common carcinogenic environmental factors that also trigger concomitant autoimmune reactions

Immune reactions against the tumor that lead to immunologic attack due to cross-reactivity with skin and muscle antigens.[50]

Tissue expression profiles have focused on common autoantigen expression and immune targeting between cancer tissue and muscle tissue in myositis.[51] Similarly, the following observations support the hypothesis that immune responses generated against myositis antigens may be related to antitumor responses:

Both DM and PM have been associated with cancer

The temporal relationship of cancer and myositis including DM/PM preceding the diagnosis of cancer

An association with specific cancer histologies

An association with distinct autoantibody profiles

The treatment of cancer mitigating the activity of myositis.

Casciola-Rosen and colleagues[52] focused their work on myositis-specific antigen expression in muscle and associated cancers to further explore this hypothesis. They showed that Mi-2 and histidyl transfer RNA synthetase (Jo-1), ubiquitously expressed in normal tissue, were increased many fold in myositis muscle tissue. Further, immunohistochemical analysis among the muscle tissue demonstrated the greatest antigen expression in the most damaged and regenerating muscle fibers. Moreover, in a model of muscle differentiation, myositis-specific autoantigens were expressed at their highest levels in immature myoblasts. They further showed that myositis-specific antigen expression was increased in random muscle biopsies of several cancer types (breast, lung) known to be associated with the development of myositis, but not in the corresponding nonmuscular tissues. By extension, these findings suggest that certain tumors and diseased/regenerating muscle are antigenic mimickers. Based on the previously mentioned studies, the authors proposed a potential mechanism for the development of CAM; increased myositis autoantigen expression in a nascent tumor leads to the generation of T and B cells directed against those antigens with subsequent successful tumor immunity. In a subset of patients, a second factor, perhaps environmental, (ie, viral infection, trauma, toxin exposure) results in muscle damage and increased expression of myositis-specific autoantigens, which recapitulate immune responses previously generated in the initial antitumor response. This hypothesis was further supported by the report of autoantibodies to PMS1 antigen (DNA mismatch repair protein) in 8 patients with pancreatic adenocarcinoma with PMS1 expression increased in affected tissue.[53] PMS1 is a known myositis-associated autoantigen, and pancreatic cancer is strongly associated with DM.

Several reports describe marked improvement in myositis signs and symptoms after chemotherapy or tumor resection,[54–56] suggesting that a decreased tumor burden mitigates the autoimmune response by decreasing the autoantigen burden to subthreshold levels. Perhaps most myositis patients not developing CAM (approximately 80%) never develop overt malignancy due to successful tumor immunity. Immune recognition of the different epitopes of the Mi-2 antigen supports the concept that patients with CAM may target different epitopes of commonly targeted autoantigens (eg, Mi-2) as opposed to IIM patients without cancer.[57] The aforementioned hypothesis, although plausible, raises additional questions as to why crossover immunity only occurs in the minority of patients developing CAM, whereas most patients feature either a malignant or autoimmune phenotype. Similarly, the genetic and environmental contributions to the ultimate expression of the mixed phenotype remain to be elucidated. Zampieri hypothesized that in genetically predisposed patients, cancer is accompanied by a subclinical tumor-induced myopathy that can later evolve to full-blown autoimmune myositis.[58] Muscle biopsies in 13 patients with myositis (3 with CAM) were compared with 14 patients with colorectal cancer unrelated to myositis and 19 healthy controls. The muscle biopsy findings in the colorectal cancer patients were similar to the histopathological features observed in the muscle from myositis patients, especially CAM, showing internally nucleated and regenerating myofibers, most of which expressed the neural cell adhesion molecule. These findings are intriguing but nonspecific. Genetic studies on CAM are limited. Andras conducted genetic studies in 145 patients with DM/PM, 10 of whom had CAM, but no HLA associations were found in the CAM patients.[9] Animal models of malignancy demonstrating some or all of the features discussed previously are necessary to elucidate the enigmatic immunopathogenic mechanisms of cancer-associated myositis.

SCREENING FOR CANCER IN PATIENTS WITH MYOSITIS

It is widely accepted that the presence of malignancy is a poor prognostic indicator in DM and PM. There are two different approaches regarding the extent of diagnostic investigating for an occult malignancy in these patients. One proposal is restricted to a complete history and physical examination, age-appropriate screening of malignancies, routine blood tests (complete blood count, erythrocyte sedimentation rate, complete metabolic profile), urine studies (urine analysis or cytology), fecal occult blood, chest radiograph, and any additional studies based on specific symptoms or signs. The other approach includes these studies along with a more extensive search for malignancy regardless of whether there are other clinical signs and symptoms. This would include thoraco-abdominal-pelvic computed tomography (CT) or positron emission tomography (PET) scans, gastrointestinal (GI) and bronchial tree endoscopic explorations, serum immunoelectrophoresis, serum tumor markers, and even bone marrow examination. The approach chosen and the optimal interval for repeating studies are controversial, with no consensus that has been decided given the lack of prospective studies. Comprehensive cancer searches require potentially invasive screening procedures, so clear and reliable methods to predict those patients with myositis at greatest risk of developing CAM are necessary. Effective screening of IIM patients could allow for early identification of cancers, and successful anticancer treatments may result in better outcomes in CAM.[1] Moreover, death in CAM almost always results from progression of malignant disease and not myositis, even in cases where the DM or PM is poorly controlled.

Early published data[59–62] did not support the usefulness of an extensive malignancy evaluation in otherwise asymptomatic patients with DM or PM. Moreover, routine malignancy screening did not enable the detection of malignancies at an early, potentially treatable stage.[63–65] To further address these questions, Sparsa retrospectively compared the usefulness of routine cancer screening versus extensive screening in a cohort of 40 adult myositis patients (16 with CAM; 3/7 PM and 13/33 DM). The rate of positive results was 54% (19 of 35) for routine clinically directed screens and 13% (11 of 87) for additional tests with no clinical indication. Thoraco-abdominal-pelvic CT scans were the most useful blind examinations, accounting for 28% (5 of 18) of the positive results. The authors proposed nondirected thoracoabdominal CT scans in men and thoracoabdominal–pelvic scanning in women as part of the routine testing in PM and DM patients. Although helpful in some patients, this study was limited by its small sample size, retrospective nature and lack of regression analysis.[22] Their results are similar to others that recommend DM patients undergo thoracoabdomino–pelvic CT scans in view of the notably increased risk of non-Hodgkin lymphoma, ovarian, lung, and pancreatic cancer.[2] A recent prospective study showed high sensitivity (78%), specificity (96%), PPV (78%), NPV (95%) and overall high diagnostic utility (93%) of extensive and comprehensive cancer screening, which included a complete physical examination, laboratory tests (as listed previously) thoracoabdominal CT scans, tumor markers (CA-125, CA-19-9, carcinoembryonic antigen [CEA], prostate-specific antigen), and gynecologic examination in women including pelvic ultrasonography and mammography.[66] However, no comparisons with standard screening procedures were reported in this study.

All authors recommend cancer screening that is specific for the patient's diagnosis, age, gender, ethnic background, and geographic area. For example, given that colon cancer is common in patients with DM aged over 65 years, colonoscopy may be specifically indicated in this patient group.[67] For patients with PM, chest radiography and urinary cytology might be performed at the time of diagnosis, targeting the commonest cancers in this cohort (ie, lung, bladder and non-Hodgkin lymphoma).[2] Ovarian carcinoma is overrepresented in women with DM and may be difficult to detect, requiring more sophisticated imaging techniques such as CT scans or ultrasound as well as gynecologic examination. In nonwhite patients (eg, Southeast Asians) where the risk of nasopharyngeal carcinoma is increased, appropriate cancer screening may be required.[10,14,19,20,68] As cancer risk in DM remains high for at least 3 years, and possibly 5 years after diagnosis, continued surveillance is required. In PM continued surveillance for 1 to 2 years may be sufficient.[67] Even if mortality is not prevented or survival is not prolonged for these malignant diseases, disability from myositis could be mitigated if cancers are detected and treated early. Careful evaluation of risk factors of CAM might help clinicians decide the extent of screening required in specific patients.

Regardless of the frequency and completeness of the malignancy search, cancer may unexpectedly arise in some cases. The earlier immunopathogenic hypothesis proposed by Casciola-Rosen may explain why intensive screening fails to detect the presence of malignancy (ie, remaining subclinical and contained by an immune response), and its subsequent and unpredictable presentation when the immune response fails to keep the malignancy in check.[52]

Tumor Markers in the Detection of CAM

The value of tumor markers in cancer screening of the general population is not generally recommended. However, given the higher incidence of malignancy observed in DM/PM patients, the role of these tumor makers in screening these patients is worthy of discussion. Few studies have evaluated the usefulness of tumor markers for the detection of solid tumors in CAM. Amoura assessed the diagnostic value of several circulating tumor markers for the detection of solid cancers in IIM patients.[69] One-hundred and two patients underwent extensive cancer screen at baseline consisting of thoracoabdominal–pelvic CT scans, upper and lower GI endoscopy, and a standard tumor marker panel including CEA, CA-125, and CA-19-9. Over the 5-year follow-up period, cancer developed in approximately 10% of the cohort. An elevated CA-125 level at myositis diagnosis was associated with a markedly increased risk of developing a malignancy during the follow-up period (OR 29.7, P<.0001, 95% C.I. 8.2–106.6), and for CA 19-9 there was a trend toward significance (P = .07; OR, 4.5; 95% CI, 1–18.7). This suggested that certain tumor markers might be useful in predicting an occult malignancy. Five out of the 8 patients with an elevated CA-125 at baseline developed cancer (cholangiocarcinoma, lung adenocarcinoma, rectal adenocarcinoma, papillary, and ovarian) as compared with 5 of 92 patients without an elevated CA-125. Similarly, 3 of 11 patients with an elevated CA-19-9 developed cancer, as compared with 7 of 89 patients without an elevated CA19-9 developing cancer. Furthermore, diagnostic values of elevated CA-125 and CA19-9 at screening increased when the study analysis was restricted to patients who developed a cancer within 1 year (P<.0001 and P = .018, respectively) or to patients without interstitial lung disease. Moreover, on longitudinal assessment of these tumor markers, patients with cancer had worsening or persistent increases in the levels of these markers, while patients without cancer had markers that returned to the normal range on subsequent testing. The authors recommended the routine use of cancer antigen testing using CA-125 and CA-19-9 for assessing the risk of developing cancer in PM and DM patients, especially in those without ILD.[69]

However, false positivity and nonspecific elevation of these markers in benign conditions raise some concerns about their routine usefulness. In a smaller sample, Whitmore showed that CA-125 was elevated several months before the diagnosis of ovarian cancer in 2 of 4 DM cases as compared with 0 of 10 DM controls without ovarian cancer. The sensitivity of CA-125 in their study was 50%, but specificity was 100% (relative risk 20, 95% C.I. [0.64, 666]).[70] Currently, CA-125 screening is not recommended as a screening tool for ovarian cancer in the general population due to its low sensitivity and low PPV for detecting early disease. However, in contrast to the population at large, females with DM may represent a unique subgroup as they are at increased risk for having nonmucinous epithelial ovarian cancer, for which the sensitivities of CA-125 for stage 1 and stage 2 cancer are 46% and 92%, respectively.[71] Given that screening for CAM is recommended up to 5 years after the diagnosis of myositis, serial CA-125 determinations (and perhaps pelvic ultrasound or CT scans) in high-risk females patients might be useful and cost-effective despite the confounding presence of false positivity.

Whole-body PET/CT Scans in Screening of CAM

PET/CT using [18F] fluorodeoxyglucose (FDG) is one of the most sensitive imaging techniques for detecting malignant lesions, and it has been used with variable success in paraneoplastic conditions such as neurologic disorders.[72] Until recently, only small retrospective case series or sporadic case reports related to the use of PET/CT in myositis had been reported.[72–74] In a prospective 3-year multicenter study, the value of whole-body PET/CT for diagnosing occult malignancy was compared with conventional cancer screening in 55 consecutive DM/PM patients. Conventional screening included a complete physical examination and routine laboratory tests, thoracoabdominal CT scans, tumor markers (CEA, CA-125, CA-19-9, PSA), and gynecologic examination in women including ultrasonography and mammography. The authors found a similar predictive value of 93% with the 2 approaches and equivalent sensitivity, specificity, PPV, and NPV for excluding occult malignancy. Although there was no added benefit of PET/CT over conventional screening, the authors concluded that

PET/CT is comparable to broad and extensive cancer screening in terms of accuracy, and has the advantage that a single imaging test would likely be more convenient for patients. Based on these results and the high NPV of anti-p155 autoantibodies, the authors proposed yearly PET/CT scans on DM patients with positive anti-p155 auto-antibodies and PET/CT scans only at diagnosis for patients with a negative anti-p155 autoantibody.[49]

SUMMARY

There are several key observations on paraneoplastic myopathies:

The risk of cancer associated with DM is very high, whereas risk of cancer associated with PM is mildly increased

Most cancers develop within one year of the onset of myositis, although the risk remains high up to 5 years after diagnosis.

The most common cancers associated with DM are adenocarcinoma, including lung, ovary, cervical, stomach, pancreas, colorectal and lymphoma, whereas PM is associated with a high risk of lymphoma.

The clinical course of myopathy is closely linked with the course of cancer.

Certain clinical features are associated with CAM including severe treatment-resistant skin manifestations, severe muscle weakness, respiratory muscle weakness, and dysphagia, while some clinical features are protective such as arthritis, Raynaud, and ILD.

Screening should be based on age, gender, ethnicity, and the geographic area of the patient; however, certain high-risk patients may require more extensive screening including tumor markers and thoracoabdominal–pelvic CT scans.

Certain autoantibodies including anti-p155 and the absence of more common autoantibodies are associated with a higher risk of CAM, while the presence of antisynthetase autoantibodies lowers the risk for CAM.

Although the pathogenesis of CAM is unclear, a plausible hypothesis is that immune responses generated against antigens commonly targeted in myositis are related to antitumor responses in affected individuals.

REFERENCES

1. Buchbinder R, Forbes A, Hall S, et al. Incidence of malignant disease in biopsy-proven inflammatory myopathy. A population-based cohort study. Ann Intern Med 2001;134(12):1087–95.
2. Hill CL, Zhang Y, Sigurgeirsson B, et al. Frequency of specific cancer types in dermatomyositis and polymyositis: a population-based study. Lancet 2001; 357(9250):96–100.
3. Sigurgeirsson B, Lindelof B, Edhag O, et al. Risk of cancer in patients with dermatomyositis or polymyositis. A population-based study. N Engl J Med 1992; 326(6):363–7.
4. Stockton D, Doherty VR, Brewster DH. Risk of cancer in patients with dermatomyositis or polymyositis, and follow-up implications: a Scottish population-based cohort study. Br J Cancer 2001;85(1):41–5.
5. Zantos D, Zhang Y, Felson D. The overall and temporal association of cancer with polymyositis and dermatomyositis. J Rheumatol 1994;21(10):1855–9.
6. Chow WI I, Gridley G, Mellemkjaer L, et al. Cancer risk following polymyositis and dermatomyositis: a nationwide cohort study in Denmark. Cancer Causes Control 1995;6(1):9–13.

7. Antiochos BB, Brown LA, Li Z, et al. Malignancy is associated with dermatomyositis but not polymyositis in Northern New England, USA. J Rheumatol 2009; 36(12):2704–10.

8. Airio A, Pukkala E, Isomaki H. Elevated cancer incidence in patients with dermatomyositis: a population-based study. J Rheumatol 1995;22(7):1300–3.

9. Andras C, Ponyi A, Constantin T, et al. Dermatomyositis and polymyositis associated with malignancy: a 21-year retrospective study. J Rheumatol 2008;35(3): 438–44.

10. Chen YJ, Wu CY, Shen JL. Predicting factors of malignancy in dermatomyositis and polymyositis: a case–control study. Br J Dermatol 2001;144(4):825–31.

11. Chinoy H, Fertig N, Oddis CV, et al. The diagnostic utility of myositis autoantibody testing for predicting the risk of cancer-associated myositis. Ann Rheum Dis 2007;66(10):1345–9.

12. Wakata N, Kurihara T, Saito E, et al. Polymyositis and dermatomyositis associated with malignancy: a 30-year retrospective study. Int J Dermatol 2002;41(11): 729–34.

13. Lee SW, Jung SY, Park MC, et al. Malignancies in Korean patients with inflammatory myopathy. Yonsei Med J 2006;47(4):519–23.

14. Peng JC, Sheen TS, Hsu MM. Nasopharyngeal carcinoma with dermatomyositis. Analysis of 12 cases. Arch Otolaryngol Head Neck Surg 1995;121(11): 1298–301.

15. Chen YJ, Wu CY, Huang YL, et al. Cancer risks of dermatomyositis and polymyositis: a nationwide cohort study in Taiwan. Arthritis Res Ther 2010;12(2):R70.

16. Callen JP. Relationship of cancer to inflammatory muscle diseases. Dermatomyositis, polymyositis, and inclusion body myositis. Rheum Dis Clin North Am 1994; 20(4):943–53.

17. Rider LG, Feldman BM, Perez MD, et al. Development of validated disease activity and damage indices for the juvenile idiopathic inflammatory myopathies: I. Physician, parent, and patient global assessments. Juvenile Dermatomyositis Disease Activity Collaborative Study Group. Arthritis Rheum 1997;40(11): 1976–83.

18. Whitmore SE, Watson R, Rosenshein NB, et al. Dermatomyositis sine myositis: association with malignancy. J Rheumatol 1996;23(1):101–5.

19. Ang P, Sugeng MW, Chua SH. Classical and amyopathic dermatomyositis seen at the National Skin Centre of Singapore: a 3-year retrospective review of their clinical characteristics and association with malignancy. Ann Acad Med Singap 2000;29(2):219–23.

20. Fung WK, Chan HL, Lam WM. Amyopathic dermatomyositis in Hong Kong—association with nasopharyngeal carcinoma. Int J Dermatol 1998;37(9):659–63.

21. Gerami P, Schope JM, McDonald L, et al. A systematic review of adult-onset clinically amyopathic dermatomyositis (dermatomyositis sine myositis): a missing link within the spectrum of the idiopathic inflammatory myopathies. J Am Acad Dermatol 2006;54(4):597–613.

22. Sparsa A, Liozon E, Herrmann F, et al. Routine vs extensive malignancy search for adult dermatomyositis and polymyositis: a study of 40 patients. Arch Dermatol 2002;138(7):885–90.

23. Selva-O'Callaghan A, Mijares-Boeckh-Behrens T, Solans-Laque R, et al. The neural network as a predictor of cancer in patients with inflammatory myopathies. Arthritis Rheum 2002;46(9):2547–8.

24. Gallais V, Crickx B, Belaich S. Prognostic factors and predictive signs of malignancy in adult dermatomyositis. Ann Dermatol Venereol 1996;123(11):722–6.

25. Basset-Seguin N, Roujeau JC, Gherardi R, et al. Prognostic factors and predictive signs of malignancy in adult dermatomyositis. A study of 32 cases. Arch Dermatol 1990;126(5):633–7.

26. Hunger RE, Durr C, Brand CU. Cutaneous leukocytoclastic vasculitis in dermatomyositis suggests malignancy. Dermatology 2001;202(2):123–6.

27. Rider LG, Miller FW. Idiopathic inflammatory muscle disease: clinical aspects. Baillieres Best Pract Res Clin Rheumatol 2000;14(1):37–54.

28. Ponyi A, Constantin T, Garami M, et al. Cancer-associated myositis: clinical features and prognostic signs. Ann N Y Acad Sci 2005;1051:64–71.

29. Fardet L, Dupuy A, Gain M, et al. Factors associated with underlying malignancy in a retrospective cohort of 121 patients with dermatomyositis. Medicine 2009; 88(2):91–7.

30. Love LA, Leff RL, Fraser DD, et al. A new approach to the classification of idiopathic inflammatory myopathy: myositis-specific autoantibodies define useful homogeneous patient groups. Medicine (Baltimore) 1991;70(6):360–74.

31. Miller FW. Myositis-specific autoantibodies. Touchstones for understanding the inflammatory myopathies. JAMA 1993;270(15):1846–9.

32. Rozelle A, Trieu S, Chung L. Malignancy in the setting of the antisynthetase syndrome. J Clin Rheumatol 2008;14(5):285–8.

33. Watkins J, Farzaneh-Far R, Tahir H, et al. Jo-1 syndrome with associated poorly differentiated adenocarcinoma. Rheumatology 2004;43(3):389–90.

34. Legault D, McDermott J, Crous-Tsanaclis AM, et al. Cancer-associated myositis in the presence of anti-Jo1 autoantibodies and the antisynthetase syndrome. J Rheumatol 2008;35(1):169–71.

35. Douglas WW, Tazelaar HD, Hartman TE, et al. Polymyositis–dermatomyositis-associated interstitial lung disease. Am J Respir Crit Care Med 2001;164(7):1182–5.

36. Hidano A, Torikai S, Uemura T, et al. Malignancy and interstitial pneumonitis as fatal complications in dermatomyositis. J Dermatol 1992;19(3):153–60.

37. Naschitz JE, Rosner I, Rozenbaum M, et al. Rheumatic syndromes: clues to occult neoplasia. Semin Arthritis Rheum 1999;29(1):43–55.

38. Selva-O'Callaghan A, Fonollosa-Pla V, Trallero-Araguas E, et al. Nailfold capillary microscopy in adults with inflammatory myopathy. Semin Arthritis Rheum 2010; 39(5):398–404.

39. Amato AA, Barohn RJ. Evaluation and treatment of inflammatory myopathies. J Neurol Neurosurg Psychiatr 2009;80(10):1060–8.

40. Trallero-Araguas E, Labrador-Horrillo M, Selva-O'Callaghan A, et al. Cancer-associated myositis and anti-p155 autoantibody in a series of 85 patients with idiopathic inflammatory myopathy. Medicine 2010;89(1):47–52.

41. Seelig HP, Moosbrugger I, Ehrfeld H, et al. The major dermatomyositis-specific Mi-2 autoantigen is a presumed helicase involved in transcriptional activation. Arthritis Rheum 1995;38(10):1389–99.

42. Zhang Y, LeRoy G, Seelig HP, et al. The dermatomyositis-specific autoantigen Mi2 is a component of a complex containing histone deacetylase and nucleosome remodeling activities. Cell 1998;95(2):279–89.

43. O'Hanlon TP, Carrick DM, Targoff IN, et al. Immunogenetic risk and protective factors for the idiopathic inflammatory myopathies: distinct HLA-A, -B, -Cw, -DRB1, and -DQA1 allelic profiles distinguish European American patients with different myositis autoantibodies. Medicine 2006;85(2):111–27.

44. Hengstman GJ, ter Laak HJ, Vree Egberts WT, et al. Anti-signal recognition particle autoantibodies: marker of a necrotising myopathy. Ann Rheum Dis 2006;65(12):1635–8.

45. Targoff IN, Mamyrova G, Trieu EP, et al. A novel autoantibody to a 155-kd protein is associated with dermatomyositis. Arthritis Rheum 2006;54(11):3682–9.
46. Kaji K, Fujimoto M, Hasegawa M, et al. Identification of a novel autoantibody reactive with 155 and 140 kDa nuclear proteins in patients with dermatomyositis: an association with malignancy. Rheumatology 2007;46(1):25–8.
47. Fujikawa K, Kawakami A, Kaji K, et al. Association of distinct clinical subsets with myositis-specific autoantibodies towards anti-155/140-kDa polypeptides, anti-140-kDa polypeptides, and antiaminoacyl tRNA synthetases in Japanese patients with dermatomyositis: a single-centre, cross-sectional study. Scand J Rheumatol 2009;38(4):263–7.
48. Gunawardena H, Wedderburn LR, North J, et al. Clinical associations of autoantibodies to a p155/140 kDa doublet protein in juvenile dermatomyositis. Rheumatology 2008;47(3):324–8.
49. Selva-O'Callaghan A, Trallero-Araguas E, Grau-Junyent JM, et al. Malignancy and myositis: novel autoantibodies and new insights. Curr Opin Rheumatol 2010;22(6):627–32.
50. Bonnetblanc JM, Bernard P, Fayol J. Dermatomyositis and malignancy. A multicenter cooperative study. Dermatologica 1990;180(4):212–6.
51. Levine SM. Cancer and myositis: new insights into an old association. Curr Opin Rheumatol 2006;18(6):620–4.
52. Casciola-Rosen L, Nagaraju K, Plotz P, et al. Enhanced autoantigen expression in regenerating muscle cells in idiopathic inflammatory myopathy. J Exp Med 2005; 201(4):591–601.
53. Casciola-Rosen LA, Pluta AF, Plotz PH, et al. The DNA mismatch repair enzyme PMS1 is a myositis-specific autoantigen. Arthritis Rheum 2001;44(2): 389–96.
54. Tallai B, Flasko T, Gyorgy T, et al. Prostate cancer underlying acute, definitive dermatomyositis: successful treatment with radical perineal prostatectomy. Clin Rheumatol 2006;25(1):119–20.
55. Yoshinaga A, Hayashi T, Ishii N, et al. Successful cure of dermatomyositis after treatment of nonseminomatous testicular cancer. Int J Urol 2005;12(6):593–5.
56. Masuda H, Urushibara M, Kihara K. Successful treatment of dermatomyositis associated with adenocarcinoma of the prostate after radical prostatectomy. J Urol 2003;169(3):1084.
57. Hengstman GJ, Vree Egberts WT, Seelig HP, et al. Clinical characteristics of patients with myositis and autoantibodies to different fragments of the Mi-2 beta antigen. Ann Rheum Dis 2006;65(2):242–5.
58. Zampieri S, Valente M, Adami N, et al. Polymyositis, dermatomyositis and malignancy: a further intriguing link. Autoimmun Rev 2010;9(6):449–53.
59. Callen JP, Hyla JF, Bole GG Jr, et al. The relationship of dermatomyositis and polymyositis to internal malignancy. Arch Dermatol 1980;116(3):295–8.
60. Callen JP. The value of malignancy evaluation in patients with dermatomyositis. J Am Acad Dermatol 1982;6(2):253–9.
61. Callen JP. Malignancy in polymyositis/dermatomyositis. Clin Dermatol 1988;6(2): 55–63.
62. Richardson JB, Callen JP. Dermatomyositis and malignancy. Med Clin North Am 1989;73(5):1211–20.
63. Schulman P, Kerr LD, Spiera H. A reexamination of the relationship between myositis and malignancy. J Rheumatol 1991;18(11):1689–92.
64. Whitmore SE, Rosenshein NB, Provost TT. Ovarian cancer in patients with dermatomyositis. Medicine 1994;73(3):153–60.

65. Davis MD, Ahmed I. Ovarian malignancy in patients with dermatomyositis and polymyositis: a retrospective analysis of fourteen cases. J Am Acad Dermatol 1997;37:730–3.
66. Selva-O'Callaghan A, Grau JM, Gamez-Cenzano C, et al. Conventional cancer screening versus PET/CT in dermatomyositis/polymyositis. Am J Med 2010; 123(6):558–62.
67. Marie I, Hatron PY, Levesque H, et al. Influence of age on characteristics of polymyositis and dermatomyositis in adults. Medicine 1999;78(3):139–47.
68. Leow YH, Goh CL. Malignancy in adult dermatomyositis. Int J Dermatol 1997; 36(12):904–7.
69. Amoura Z, Duhaut P, Huong DL, et al. Tumor antigen markers for the detection of solid cancers in inflammatory myopathies. Cancer Epidemiol Biomarkers Prev 2005;14(5):1279–82.
70. Whitmore SE, Anhalt GJ, Provost TT, et al. Serum CA-125 screening for ovarian cancer in patients with dermatomyositis. Gynecol Oncol 1997;65(2):241–4.
71. Carlson KJ, Skates SJ, Singer DE. Screening for ovarian cancer. Ann Intern Med 1994;121(2):124–32.
72. McKeon A, Apiwattanakul M, Lachance DH, et al. Positron emission tomography–computed tomography in paraneoplastic neurologic disorders: systematic analysis and review. Arch Neurol 2010;67(3):322–9.
73. Liau N, Ooi C, Reid C, et al. F-18 FDG PET/CT detection of mediastinal malignancy in a patient with dermatomyositis. Clin Nucl Med 2007;32(4):304–5.
74. Kim HS, Kim CH, Park YH, et al. 18Fluorine fluorodeoxyglucose-positron emission tomography/computed tomography in dermatomyositis. Joint Bone Spine 2008; 75(4):508–10.

Neoplasm Mimics of Rheumatologic Presentations: Sialadenitis, Ocular Masquerade Syndromes, Retroperitoneal Fibrosis, and Regional Pain Syndromes

Sarah Lipton, MD, Pascale Schwab, MD*

KEYWORDS

- Cancer • Sialadenitis • IgG4-related syndrome
- Ocular masquerade syndrome • Retroperitoneal fibrosis
- Complex regional pain syndrome • Amyloidosis

In their assessment of undiagnosed systemic diseases or unusual regional pain syndromes, rheumatologists should consider a broad differential diagnosis beyond the common rheumatologic conditions and particularly evaluate for the possibility of an occult malignancy. Other articles in this issue focus on specific rheumatologic presentations of cancer. This article reviews a heterogeneous group of disorders not included elsewhere in this issue, including sialadenitis, ocular masquerade syndromes, retroperitoneal fibrosis, complex regional pain syndrome, and entrapment neuropathy. These conditions may present to the rheumatologist because of features shared with common systemic inflammatory conditions or regional rheumatologic syndromes, but may be the result of a solid tumor or a lymphoproliferative disease.

The authors have no financial disclosures.
Division of Arthritis and Rheumatic Diseases, Oregon Health and Science University, Portland Veterans Affairs Medical Center, 3181 SW Sam Jackson Park Road, OP09, Portland, OR 97239, USA
* Corresponding author.
E-mail address: schwabp@ohsu.edu

SALIVARY GLAND ENLARGEMENT AND DYSFUNCTION

In their evaluation of salivary gland enlargement and dysfunction, rheumatologists should not only consider Sjögren syndrome but also lymphoproliferative disorders such as immunoglobulin (Ig) G4–related systemic disease (IgG4-RSD) and malignancy.

Sjögren Syndrome

Sjögren syndrome is an autoimmune-mediated inflammation of the lacrimal and salivary glands that rheumatologists are frequently asked to evaluate; in these cases, the entire differential diagnosis must be considered, including malignant or lymphoproliferative processes. Ocular and oral dryness are common symptoms, particularly in elderly patients who frequently experience glandular age-related atrophy. Other common causes of ocular dryness include anticholinergic drugs, nonautoimmune gland dysfunction from blepharitis, or mechanical factors.[1] Likewise, oral sicca may be caused by medications or chronic viral infections such as human immunodeficiency virus (HIV) and hepatitis C,[2] following radiation therapy, as part of graft-versus-host disease, or as a result of infiltrative diseases such as sarcoidosis.[3] Sjögren syndrome is characterized by lymphocytic infiltration, enlargement, and dysfunction of glandular tissue and is associated with the presence of antinuclear antibodies, anti-Ro and anti-La antibodies, rheumatoid factor, as well as extraglandular features in 25% and lymphoma in 2.5%.[4] It is primary in 70% of cases or otherwise secondary to rheumatoid arthritis and other connective tissue diseases.[5] The histology of Sjögren syndrome is coined benign lymphoepithelial sialadenitis (also known as myoepithelial sialadenitis [MESA]). Pathologic features include lymphocytic infiltration, parenchymal atrophy, and foci of epithelial proliferation. These findings may be localized initially, but, late in the disease, may involve the entire gland while preserving its architecture. Ductal hyperplasia, together with foci of lymphocyte infiltration, constitutes the lymphoepithelial lesion and results in ductal luminal obliteration.[6] T cells (with occasional B cells) primarily constitute the lymphoid infiltrate. B cell clonal expansion is found in 50% of MESA by molecular genetics.[7] Although, in some cases, this may represent the earliest manifestation of lymphoma,[8] much uncertainty regarding this continuum remains,[9] and malignant progression may require additional oncogenic mutations.[10] A high index of suspicion for the development of salivary gland lymphoma should be maintained for the lifetime of a patient with Sjögren syndrome.[11]

Salivary Gland Lymphoma

Salivary gland lymphomas represent 1.7% to 7% of all salivary gland tumors and are usually primary and only rarely secondary to extraglandular nodal disease. The characteristic patient is a woman in her 60s presenting with unilateral glandular enlargement. Although patients with Sjögren syndrome have an increased risk of salivary gland lymphoma, most patients with salivary gland lymphoma do not have an underlying autoimmune disease. Most salivary gland lymphomas are non-Hodgkin B cell lymphomas, primarily extranodal marginal zone B cell lymphoma and, less commonly, follicular or diffuse large B cell lymphomas.[6] Marginal B cell lymphomas of the salivary glands are typically mucosa-associated lymphoid tissue (MALT) lymphomas. Most MALT lymphomas are associated with a predisposing factor such as infection or an autoimmune disease resulting in the formation of lymphoid tissue at sites where it is not normally present.[12] In a series of 9 salivary MALT lymphomas, half the patients had a diagnosis of Sjögren syndrome.[13] Most of the patients were women, had localized disease with good prognostic factors, and had presented with asymptomatic glandular enlargement of the parotid gland. In all cases, fine-needle aspiration and radiologic imaging were not diagnostic, only raising the suspicion for a lymphoproliferative process. Blind biopsies of parotid masses should be avoided to prevent injury to the facial nerve and avoid seeding of malignant cells. Diagnosis was established in all from surgical excision.[13] Diagnostic features of MALT include broad strands of marginal zone B cells around lymphoepithelial lesions as well as the presence of monoclonal Ig expansion by immunohistochemistry.[7] Differentiation from reactive lymphoid proliferation is difficult, especially because 20% of salivary gland MALT lymphomas are found in the setting of MESA.[6]

IgG4-RSD

In 2003, Kamisawa and colleagues[14] first recognized that autoimmune pancreatitis is characterized by infiltration with IgG4-positive plasma cells that can be detected beyond the pancreatic tissue and heralds a systemic disease, which they coined IgG4-related autoimmune disease. Since then, the field has expanded into a new concept of IgG4-RSD. IgG4-RSD can cause sialadenitis and dacryoadenitis and seems to encompass the poorly characterized old entities of Kuttner tumor and Mikulicz disease.[15]

Kuttner tumor, also known as chronic sclerosing sialadenitis, was originally described by Kuttner as a hard swelling of 1 or more submandibular glands that may also involve the parotid and minor salivary gland. Patients are often middle-aged to elderly men who present with asymptomatic enlargement of salivary glands, unilateral or bilateral, with preserved to slightly reduced salivary gland function. Researchers from Japan reported on the presence of abundant IgG4 plasma cells in 12 patients with sclerosing sialadenitis and first proposed its association with IgG4-RSD.[16] About half of these patients had extrasalivary systemic lesions with either pancreatic, lacrimal, prostate, or bile duct infiltration. More than 45% of infiltrating IgG-positive plasma cells were IgG4 positive in these patients, compared with less than 5% in sialolithiasis and Sjögren control patients. IgG4 serum levels were not measured in this series. A more recent study confirmed similar findings in a Western population of patients with chronic sclerosing sialadenitis,[17] again supporting the finding that Kuttner tumor may belong within the spectrum of IgG4-RSD. Unlike MESA, lymphoepithelial lesions are not detected in Kuttner tumor. Instead, histology reveals marked lymphoplasmacytic infiltration with large germinal centers, obliterative phlebitis, acinal atrophy, and interlobular fibrosis with activated fibroblasts.[15]

Mikulicz disease presents with bilateral and persistent enlargement of the lacrimal and salivary glands. It has been rarely reported in the Western literature since Morgan and Castleman[18] defined it as a subset of Sjögren syndrome. Differences from Sjögren syndrome include a balanced gender distribution, mild keratoconjunctivitis sicca, the lack of positive antinuclear antibody or anti-Ro/La antibodies, reported positive response to corticosteroids with recovery of glandular function, and the lack of apoptosis and acinar destruction typical of Sjögren syndrome.[19] Yamamoto and colleagues[20] reported on 7 patients meeting the definition of Mikulicz disease and described increased serum IgG4 levels and the presence of IgG4-positive plasma cells infiltrating around the acinar and ductal cells, defining a new concept of Mikulicz disease as an IgG4-related plasmacytic disease.[21] Presence of greater than 50 IgG4-positive plasma cells per high-power field and an IgG4/IgG-positive plasma cell ratio of greater than 50% have been proposed as the histologic requirement for the diagnosis of IgG4-associated sialadenitis.[15]

Chronic sclerosing dacryoadenitis secondary to infiltration of the lacrimal glands by IgG4-positive plasma cells has recently been recognized in the spectrum of IgG4-related systemic disease.[22,23] In a series reviewing 112 cases with ocular adnexal lymphoproliferative disorders, 21 patients were identified as having IgG4-positive plasma cell infiltration. Most of these patients had lacrimal gland infiltration and none had conjunctival involvement.[23] Histology of the glands was similar to that of chronic sclerosing sialadenitis of the submandibular glands with lymphoplasmacytic infiltration with lymphoid follicle formation, acinar atrophy, periductal fibrosis, and sclerosis, but lacking the obliterative phlebitis described in other organs.[22,23] Several cases of MALT lymphoma arising in a background of IgG4 plasma cell infiltrative disease have also been reported.[23,24]

The pathogenesis of IgG4-RSD is poorly understood and the role of IgG4 antibodies in the inflammatory cascade is unknown. IgG4 normally represents only 3% to 6% of total IgG and levels are tightly regulated, increasing slightly with age and male gender. IgG4 differs from other IgG subtypes. The covalent bindings of its heavy chains are loose, resulting in alterations of the Fab arm specificity and in functionally monovalent antibodies, which do not bind complements or cross-link identical antigens.[25] Tissue-infiltrating and circulating plasma cells are polyclonal and therefore not of neoplastic origin.[26] IgG4 antibodies in IgG4-RSD are not antigen specific, thus arguing against an autoimmune disease.[25] The mainstay of treatment of IgG4-RSD remains corticosteroids based on retrospective experience, with little long-term follow up.[27]

Salivary Gland Cancer

Sialadenosis or isolated salivary gland enlargement may present to the rheumatologist for evaluation of Sjögren syndrome. If unilateral, the possibility of a primary salivary gland tumor must be entertained. Salivary gland neoplasms are rare and represent about 5% of all head and neck tumors, or 0.5% of all malignancies. They typically present in the sixth decade of life and, for the most part, occur equally in men and women.[28] Eighty percent of salivary gland neoplasms arise in the parotid gland, and most of those turn out to be benign pleomorphic adenomas, which comprise 50% of all tumors, followed by papillary cystadenoma, also known as Warthin tumor.[29] The most common malignant salivary gland tumor is the mucoepidermoid carcinoma, which represents 10% of all salivary gland tumors.[30] Pathogenesis of salivary gland tumors is not well understood. Factors implicated in nonsalivary head and neck tumors, such as smoking, are not known risk factors for the development of salivary gland tumors, whereas radiation therapy seems to be. Warthin tumor is the exception because it may be multifocal and bilateral, is more common in men, and is associated with smoking.[31] Salivary gland neoplasm should be suspected in a patient presenting with an enlarging painless mass. Minor salivary gland tumors may present with a persistent oral ulceration. Evaluation should include imaging with ultrasound, computed tomography (CT), or magnetic resonance imaging (MRI) to assess disease extent and guide fine-needle aspiration biopsy[32] and help plan surgical excision, which is required for accurate diagnosis and management. Prognosis of malignant tumors is based primarily on tumor size, with patients with tumors less than 4 cm doing well regardless of histologic type.[28,30]

NEOPLASTIC OCULAR MASQUERADE SYNDROMES

Ocular masquerade syndromes are a group of ocular malignant disorders that can present as ocular inflammatory diseases. Ocular malignancies are rare, and neoplasms mimicking inflammatory diseases are even rarer. However, rheumatologists may be asked to help manage the immunosuppression of patients with ocular inflammation, and these conditions should be considered in patients with an atypical course or a lack of treatment response. These conditions may not only be vision threatening but also life threatening and therefore require a high index of suspicion.[33,34]

Primary Intraocular Lymphoma

Primary intraocular lymphoma (PIOL), a rare ocular neoplasm, is frequently misdiagnosed as uveitis, vitritis, or chorioretinitis, and must be suspected in patients with vitritis or posterior uveitis that is refractory to or recurs after steroid therapy. In a series of 40 patients with a uveitis masquerade syndrome, 16 had an intraocular malignancy, of which 13 were intraocular lymphoma.[35] Immunodeficiency from transplant antirejection therapy, HIV disease, or inherited immune deficiencies should raise the clinical suspicion PIOL.[36] Diagnosis was delayed from 1 to 29 months in 1 series,[37] and is challenging for several reasons: it may initially be responsive to steroid therapy; although common, central nervous system (CNS) involvement may not occur for years following initial ocular presentation, so a normal CNS evaluation does not exclude ocular lymphoma[38]; and cytologic evaluation early in the course may be unrevealing because some of the infiltrating leucocytes may be reactive to the malignant cells.[39] PIOL typically presents in the fifth to seventh decade. Ocular symptoms are present in 80%, most often blurred vision but also eye pain, floaters, or a foreign-body sensation.[38] Eighty percent of patients may present with bilateral involvement even in the absence of bilateral ocular symptoms.[39] Fundus examination reveals vitritis universally with clumps of white cells without significant anterior chamber flare,[33,37] and may be the only finding in 30%. The classic pathognomonic feature is described as round or oval, yellow-white, dome-shaped masses in the subpigment epithelial space but may also include chorioretinitis and retinal vasculitis.[40] Ocular ultrasound may help support slit lamp findings as well as detect retrobulbar involvement in some cases.[38] Fluorescein angiography may reveal granularity, blockage, and late staining at the level of the retinal pigment epithelium and, less commonly, pathognomonic hypofluorescent pigment epithelial detachment. Other features include lack of perivascular staining and lack of cystoid macular edema, as seen in the setting of other causes of vitritis.[41] Additional evaluation should include pars plana vitrectomy or chorioretinal biopsy, if necessary. These tests are more likely to be sensitive if steroids are withheld before the procedure. Non-Hodgkin B cell lymphoma is the most common type PIOL, followed by angiotropic T cell lymphoma.[40] Although only a small sample volume with a low number of malignant cells is obtained from vitrectomy, cytologic review and processing of fresh sample for immunohistochemistry and polymerase chain reaction analysis may increase the sensitivity of the test.[42] An intravitreous interleukin (IL)-10/IL-6 ratio greater than 1.0 may suggest lymphoma.[43] Head MRI and cerebrospinal fluid examination are necessary to assess for CNS involvement, which may already be present at the time of ocular presentation or may develop in up to 80% of patients. HIV testing is also essential. Intravitreally injected methotrexate and, possibly, intravitreally injected rituximab are important adjuncts to therapy.[44] Because ocular lymphoma is usually associated with disease that extends beyond the eye, systemic chemotherapy is associated with an improved progression-free survival.[37] Given its initially indolent ocular presentation and partial response to steroids, PIOL can easily be mistaken for idiopathic uveitis and must be considered and excluded before embarking on steroid-sparing immunosuppressant therapy.

Leukemia

The typical ocular manifestations of acute leukemia are described as leukemic retinopathy and orbital infiltration, but may rarely include uveitis masquerade syndrome.

Most case reports describe children presenting with anterior uveitis as a first sign of CNS or bone marrow relapse with acute lymphoblastic leukemia.[35,45]

Periocular Lymphoma

Several cases of periocular or adnexal ocular lymphoma presenting as refractory uveitis or scleritis have been reported in the literature.[46–48] Periocular lymphoma represents about 1% to 2% of all non-Hodgkin lymphomas and is primarily a disease of older adults. The orbit is most commonly involved, followed by the conjunctivae, lacrimal glands, and the eyelids. It typically presents with a painless, salmon pink, diffuse or well-defined mass associated with proptosis, visual disturbance, periorbital edema, or redness.[49] More than 70% to 90% of ocular adnexal lymphomas are primary and not secondary to systemic lymphoma.[50,51] Most are low-grade B cell–type lymphomas. The most common histologic type is the extranodal marginal zone lymphoma of MALT[50] and has been associated with cytogenetic abnormalities including trisomies and molecular translocations.[51] Chlamydia psittaci has been implicated in the pathogenesis of ocular MALT but detection rates are highly variable among geographic regions.[52] Systemic lymphoma develops in one-third of patients within 10 years, especially when the initial orbital presentation is bilateral.[49] Therefore, a thorough evaluation and ongoing vigilance are required.

Retinoblastoma

Retinoblastoma may present as orbital inflammation in a subset of children[33,34,53–56] and should be considered in the differential diagnosis of uveitis in children. Classically, retinoblastoma presents with leukocoria, strabismus, or reduced vision in children at a mean age of 18 months, with findings of a well-defined yellow-white retinal mass with evident calcifications on imaging. In a series of 1507 patients eventually diagnosed with retinoblastoma in one tertiary care center, 2% of cases presented with a diffuse infiltrative pattern mimicking ocular inflammation.[56] The mean age was 4 years. Of those patients, 9% had been referred for evaluation of uveitis. Most presented with a white hypopyon, conjunctival injection, and vitritis,[55,56] with either a lack or subtle presence of intralesional calcifications.[53] Orbital cellulitis has also been reported as an initial presentation of diffuse retinoblastoma.[54] Diagnosis should be made clinically by an experienced examiner because needle biopsy may lead to tumor cell seeding and future metastasis. Treatment consists of enucleation with or without chemotherapy.[56]

Primary Ocular Melanoma

The eye is the second most common melanoma site. Primary ocular melanoma (POM) represents about 4% of all melanomas and is the most common primary ocular malignancy in adults, primarily affecting middle-aged white patients.[57] Ninety-five percent of all ocular melanomas localize to the posterior uveal tract (ciliary body or choroid) and 5% to the iris.[58] Most cases are sporadic. Fifty percent of cases are associated with metastasis, typically to the liver, and a 50% mortality at 10 years is reported and directly correlates with initial tumor size. Treatment consists of enucleation and local irradiation.[58] Typically, POM presents with a painless mass. However, of 450 consecutive enucleations for malignant melanoma of the choroid or ciliary body, 5% initially presented with clinical signs of ocular inflammation. Close to half of those patients had episcleritis and the others had uveitis, endophthalmitis, or panophthalmitis.[59] Cases presenting as scleritis have also been reported in the literature.[60–62] These cases may initially respond to corticosteroid treatment, delaying the diagnosis. Furthermore, the choroidal mass may be plaquelike and difficult to detect.[60] A high index of suspicion and close monitoring of mass enlargement with sequential examination, fundus photography, and orbital ultrasound are therefore recommended.[60]

RETROPERITONEAL FIBROSIS

Retroperitoneal fibrosis (RF) is characterized by a proliferating fibroinflammatory mass that surrounds the abdominal aorta and the common iliac arteries, and frequently encases nearby organs (usually the ureters). RF is rare, occurring in 1 in 200,000 people. Seventy percent of cases are idiopathic (primary) and the remaining cases are secondary to other diseases or factors. About 8% to 10% of all cases are associated with malignancy.[63] Secondary RF is most commonly caused by use of medications, mainly ergot alkaloids and dopamine agonists. Infection, particularly mycobacterial, can also cause RF. Additional causes include radiotherapy and surgery. Idiopathic RF is associated with multiple autoimmune or inflammatory diseases, including autoimmune thyroid disease, systemic lupus erythematosus, rheumatoid arthritis, ankylosing spondylitis, and several vasculitides.[64]

Work in the last several years has revealed that a fraction of cases of idiopathic RF are caused by IgG4-RSD. In IgG4-RSD the retroperitoneal involvement is typically not diffuse, but manifests as inflammatory masses involving the abdominal aorta, kidneys, or ureters. These inflammatory masses consist of lymphoplasmacytic inflammation and fibrosis, with a significant proportion of plasma cells expressing IgG4. Published cases of RF caused by IgG4-RSD have shown male predominance and involvement of other organs.[65]

In most cases of RF secondary to malignancy, the fibrosis results from a robust desmoplastic response to metastatic cells within the retroperitoneum.[66] Tumors that most commonly induce this response include Hodgkin and other lymphomas, sarcomas, and numerous carcinomas (breast, lung, pancreas, stomach, colon, rectum, kidney, bladder, prostate, ovary, and cervix).[66–69] In contrast, carcinoid tumors can cause RF (and fibrosis elsewhere) without metastasizing to the retroperitoneum. The mechanism of carcinoid-related fibrosis is not well understood. Consideration has been given to the role of local serotonin levels and tachykinins in stimulating fibroblasts, but supporting data for each are limited. Multiple growth factors stimulate growth of fibroblasts in cell cultures and are being explored as possible mediators of carcinoid-related fibrosis.[70]

Diagnosing RF and distinguishing between malignant and nonmalignant causes of RF is often challenging because many of the clinical, radiographic, and even histologic features are nonspecific. The most common presenting symptoms are back, flank, and abdominal pain. Despite frequent obstruction of the ureters, renal colic is uncommon. Systemic symptoms may include weakness, nausea, fever, fatigue, and malaise. Physical examination may reveal an abdominal or rectal mass or lower-extremity edema (resulting from venous compression), but is typically not helpful. Laboratory data commonly indicate inflammation; a mild normochromic normocytic anemia and significant increases in erythrocyte sedimentation rate or C-reactive protein are expected.[71] However, because of diagnostic challenges, delay in diagnosis is common and complications frequently ensue. Ureteral obstruction leading to acute or chronic renal insufficiency is the most common and severe complication of RF.[64]

Ultrasound is useful as a first-line imaging study for RF and can be used to detect hydronephrosis. Intravenous urography may show the triad of medial deviation and external compression of the ureters along with hydronephrosis, but these findings are not specific for RF. CT and MRI are the imaging modalities of choice for evaluating the extent of RF. Advantages of MRI compared with CT are a more precise anatomic definition because of multiplanar capability and avoidance of iodinated contrast in patients with compromised renal function.[72] Malignant RF, unlike idiopathic RF, typically displaces the aorta anteriorly and the ureters laterally.[64] Lymphoma and other malignancies can cause both of those findings, but usually occur in a more cranial location. RF does not cause local bone destruction, which can occur in retroperitoneal neoplasms. MRI characteristics that suggest malignant RF include heterogeneity of the mass and higher signal intensity on T2-weighted images than on T1-weight images.[72] Although fluorodeoxyglucose-positron emission tomography (FDG-PET) is not useful in diagnosing RF because of low specificity, it can be useful in assessing metabolic activity of the retroperitoneal mass and for detecting other foci of disease (such as in malignancy, infection, and IgG4-RSD).[64]

Microscopically, RF is described as sclerotic tissue infiltrated by mononuclear cells. Inflammatory infiltrates are composed of lymphocytes (with CD20 and B cells outnumbering T cells), macrophages, plasma cells, and eosinophils. Fibroblastlike cells are also present. Although the histologic appearance of primary and secondary forms of RF are similar, in malignant RF, neoplastic cells may be detected among the fibrous tissue, and invasion or destruction of muscle and other neighboring structures may be seen.[64] It is particularly difficult to distinguish RF from sclerosing lymphomas; thorough immunohistochemical staining is crucial especially because immunomodulatory therapy used in the treatment of idiopathic RF can further mask and delay diagnosis of lymphoma.[63]

Treatment of malignant RF is directed toward the underlying malignancy.[72] If present, ureteral obstruction must also be relieved. However, malignant RF has a poor prognosis, with mean survival of 3 to 6 months following diagnosis.[72] Idiopathic RF carries a less dire prognosis when managed with medical therapy and with surgical therapy as needed.[73] Data guiding choice of therapy for idiopathic RF are limited. Corticosteroids are considered the cornerstone of medical therapy, and recent small studies suggest that mycophenolate mofetil and tamoxifen may also have a role, although further studies are warranted.[74–76]

REGIONAL PAIN SYNDROMES
Complex Regional Pain Syndrome

Complex regional pain syndrome (CRPS) is a regional, neuropathic condition of poorly understood pathogenesis that usually affects 1 or more limbs. Other names for this entity include reflex sympathetic dystrophy (RSD), causalgia, Sudek atrophy, and shoulder-hand syndrome. CRPS typically presents with burning pain, allodynia, and hyperalgesia. Sympathetic dysfunction, such as vasomotor and sudomotor instability may be observed. Joint swelling and stiffness may also be reported. Motor findings such as tremor, dystonia, and weakness may be present but are not necessary for the diagnosis. Later stages of the disease are characterized by trophic changes of nails and hair, brawny edema, and contractures that may mimic systemic sclerosis.[77,78] Patchy osteoporosis reflecting immobility and disuse may be seen on plain radiographs as early as 2 weeks into the disease course, although increased uptake on a 3-phase technetium-labeled bone scan may allow for earlier detection.[79] Additional evaluation should include efforts to rule out other conditions such as vascular occlusion and nerve entrapment. The pathophysiology of CRPS is not well understood. Several mechanisms, including neurogenic inflammation, vasomotor dysfunction, and maladaptive neuroplasticity, have been implicated.[80] Well-described inciting events include trauma (which may be minor), stroke, and myocardial infarction.[81] Although occult malignancy is not regularly included in the differential diagnosis, multiple case reports have suggested an association with CRPS. CRPS may be the initial presentation and may precede the cancer diagnosis by months.[82]

Occult neoplasms of brain, lung, breast, bowel, and ovarian origins have been reported to present with CRPS.[83] Supporting the association has been the observation that, in many cases, treatment of the underlying malignancy led to resolution of pain and improvement of range of motion.[82,84] Pancoast tumor (neoplasm of the apex of the lung) can result in CRPS by direct infiltration or entrapment of neurovascular structures that run in the superior inlet of the thorax, including the sympathetic chain, the stellate ganglion, and the brachial plexus.[85,86] Ovarian cancer has been associated with a shoulder-hand syndrome characterized by pain and limitation of range of motion of the shoulders and hands with features of polyarthritis and palmar fasciitis, and portends a particularly poor prognosis.[78,83,87] Peripheral musculoskeletal tumors, including osteoid osteoma and epithelioid sarcoma, may masquerade as CRPS in rare cases.[88,89] CRPS may also be the consequence of cancer therapy such as bone marrow transplant,[90] radical neck dissection,[91] and chemotherapy, as described with everolimus treatment of renal cell carcinoma.[92] In cancer-associated CRPS, treatment should focus on cancer cure; however, a multidisciplinary approach combining patient education, physical therapy, and pain management is the key to optimizing recovery.[81]

Amyloid Light Chain Amyloidosis and Compressive Neuropathy

The term amyloid refers to proteins that have a β-pleated sheet configuration, apple green birefringence under polarized light after Congo red staining, fibrillary structure, and high insolubility. Amyloid deposition may be localized or systemic. One form of systemic disease is amyloid light chain (AL) amyloidosis, a plasma cell dyscrasia in which amyloid is derived from immunoglobulin light chain fragments. AL amyloidosis can occur as a primary disease or as a complication of multiple myeloma, Waldenström macroglobulinemia, non-Hodgkin lymphoma, and certain solid malignancies (such as renal cell carcinoma). Primary AL amyloidosis is rare (8.9 cases per million per year), with a mean age of onset of 62 years. Many organ systems can be involved but typical locations include the tongue, heart, gastrointestinal tract, kidney, large joints, and peripheral nerves. In 80% of cases, a monoclonal (M) protein can be found in the serum or urine.[93]

Approximately 25% of patients with AL amyloidosis develop carpal tunnel syndrome caused by amyloid deposition in the flexor retinaculum of the wrist, which may occur before or after onset of more generalized illness.[94] In addition, patients with AL amyloidosis who undergo electromyographic testing for evaluation of peripheral neuropathy may be found to have median nerve compression that is asymptomatic.[95] Femoral nerve compression caused by hypertrophic amyloid myopathy has also been described in AL amyloidosis.[96]

Because carpal tunnel syndrome is common in the general population, diagnosing underlying amyloidosis may be challenging. In one series, symptoms of carpal tunnel syndrome were present for a mean duration of 19 months before diagnosis of amyloidosis.[97] Evidence of other organ involvement may be helpful in prompting further evaluation for amyloidosis in a patient who presents with carpal tunnel syndrome, because its clinical presentation and electromyographic findings are nonspecific.[98] Although detecting a serum or urine monoclonal protein is an important step in diagnosis, obtaining tissue (via an involved organ or a surrogate site such as abdominal fat) and showing and typing amyloid are essential for diagnosis and choice of therapy.

Extent of organ involvement must be determined, with special attention to cardiac assessment as, because myocardial disease carries a particularly poor prognosis.[99]

Median survival of untreated AL amyloidosis is 12 months.[99] The goal of treatment is eliminating the supply of newly formed light chains; rapid initiation of treatment is imperative in preventing or reversing organ damage. In recent years, choices for therapy have greatly expanded. The 2 most widely used treatment regimens are MDex (melphalan and high-dose dexamethasone) and SCT (high-dose melphalan followed by rescue with autologous stem cell transplantation). Measurement of free light chain concentration, along with sensitive cardiac biomarkers when the heart is involved, is useful in monitoring response to therapy.[100]

SUMMARY

IgG4-RSD should be suspected in any patient presenting with lacrimal or salivary gland enlargement, particularly if male and manifesting mild glandular dysfunction. A serum IgG4 level, if increased, may be helpful, although a gland biopsy staining for IgG4-positive plasma cells is the definitive test. Primary low-grade B cell lymphomas of the glandular tissue, specifically MALT lymphoma and other glandular malignancy, should be considered, particularly in patients with asymmetric glandular enlargement. Patients with idiopathic uveitis should have a thorough evaluation to exclude malignancy, in particular PIOL and melanoma in adults, and diffuse retinoblastoma and ALL in children. RF remains a diagnostic challenge and atypical features such as outward displacement of the retroperitoneal structures should raise the suspicion for a malignant infiltrative process. CRPS rarely may be the first presentation of an occult malignancy and requires a thorough review of age-appropriate cancer screening. Carpal tunnel syndrome, if bilateral or associated with other systemic features, should prompt a search for amyloidosis.

ACKNOWLEDGMENTS

We appreciate Jim Rosenbaum's helpful comments and review of the manuscript.

REFERENCES

1. Schein OD, Hochberg MC, Munoz B, et al. Dry eye and dry mouth in the elderly: a population-based assessment. Arch Intern Med 1999;159(12):1359–63.
2. Ramos-Casals M, Font J. Extrahepatic manifestations in patients with chronic hepatitis C virus infection. Curr Opin Rheumatol 2005;17(4):447–55.
3. Ramos-Casals M, Brito-Zeron P, Garcia-Carrasco M, et al. Sarcoidosis or Sjogren syndrome? Clues to defining mimicry or coexistence in 59 cases. Medicine (Baltimore) 2004;83(2):85–9.
4. Asmussen K, Andersen V, Bendixen G, et al. A new model classification of disease manifestations in primary Sjogren's syndrome: evaluation in a retrospective long-term study. J Intern Med 1996;239(6):475–82.
5. Fox RI, Stern M, Michelson P. Upgrade in Sjogren syndrome. Curr Opin Rheumatol 2000;12(5):391–8.
6. Ellis GL. Lymphoid lesions of salivary glands: malignant and benign. Med Oral Patol Oral Cir Bucal 2007;12(7):E479–85.
7. Harris NL. Lymphoid proliferations of the salivary glands. Am J Clin Pathol 1999; 111(1 Suppl 1):S94–103.

8. Falzon M, Isaacson PG. The natural history of benign lymphoepithelial lesion of the salivary gland in which there is a monoclonal population of B cells. A report of 2 cases. Am J Surg Pathol 1991;15(1):59–65.

9. Youinou P, Devauchelle-Pensec V, Pers JO. Significance of B cells and B cell clonality in Sjogren syndrome. Arthritis Rheum 2010;62(9):2605–10.

10. Bahler DW, Swerdlow SH. Clonal salivary gland infiltrates associated with myooepithelial sialadenitis begin as non-malignant antigen-selected expansions. Blood 1998;91(6):1864–72.

11. Mariette X. Lymphomas in patients with Sjogren's syndrome: review of the literature and physiopathologic hypothesis. Leuk Lymphoma 1999;33(1–2):93–9.

12. Isaacson PG, Du MQ. MALT lymphoma: from morphology to molecules. Nat Rev Cancer 2004;4(8):644–53.

13. Toso A, Aluffi P, Capello D, et al. Clinical and molecular features of mucosa-associated lymphoid tissue (MALT) lymphomas of salivary glands. Head Neck 2009;31(9):1181–7.

14. Kamisawa T, Funata N, Hayashi Y, et al. A new clinicopathological entity of IgG4-related autoimmune disease. J Gastroenterol 2003;38(10):982–4.

15. Geyer JT, Deshpande V. IgG4-associated sialadenitis. Curr Opin Rheumatol 2011;23(1):95–101.

16. Kitagawa S, Zen Y, Harada K, et al. Abundant IgG4-positive plasma cell infiltration characterizes chronic sclerosing sialadenitis (Kuttner's tumor). Am J Surg Pathol 2005;29(6):783–91.

17. Geyer JT, Ferry JA, Harris NL, et al. Chronic sclerosing sialadenitis (Kuttner tumor) is an IgG4-associated disease. Am J Surg Pathol 2010;34(2):202–10.

18. Morgan WS, Castleman B. A clinicopathologic study of Mikulicz's disease. Am J Pathol 1953;29(3):471–503.

19. Yamamoto M, Harada S, Ohara M, et al. Beneficial effects of steroid therapy for Mikulicz's disease. Rheumatology (Oxford) 2005;44(10):1322–3.

20. Yamamoto M, Harada S, Ohara M, et al. Clinical and pathological differences between Mikulicz's disease and Sjogren syndrome. Rheumatology (Oxford) 2005;44(2):227–34.

21. Yamamoto M, Takahashi H, Ohara M, et al. A new conceptualization for Mikulicz's disease as an IgG4-related plasmacytic disease. Mod Rheumatol 2006; 16(6):335–40.

22. Cheuk W, Yuen HK, Chan JK. Chronic sclerosing dacryoadenitis: part of the spectrum of IgG4-related sclerosing disease? Am J Surg Pathol 2007;31(4): 643–5.

23. Sato Y, Ohshima K, Ichimura K, et al. Ocular adnexal IgG4-related disease has uniform clinicopathology. Pathol Int 2008;58(8):465–70.

24. Cheuk W, Yuen HK, Chan AC, et al. Ocular adnexal lymphoma associated with IgG4+ chronic sclerosing dacryoadenitis: a previously undescribed complication of IgG4-related sclerosing disease. Am J Surg Pathol 2008;32(8):1159–67.

25. Nirula A, Glaser SM, Kalled SL, et al. What is IgG4? A review of the biology of a unique immunoglobulin subtype. Curr Opin Rheumatol 2011;23(1):119–24.

26. Yamada K, Kawano M, Inoue R, et al. Clonal relationship between infiltrating immunoglobulin G4 (IgG4)-positive plasma cells in lacrimal glands and circulating IgG4-positive lymphocytes in Mikulicz's disease. Clin Exp Immunol 2008;152(3):432–9.

27. Khosroshahi A, Stone JH. Treatment approaches to IgG4-related systemic disease. Curr Opin Rheumatol 2011;23(1):67–71.

28. Speight PM, Barrett AW. Salivary gland tumours. Oral Dis 2002;8(5):229–40.

29. Spiro RH. Salivary neoplasms: overview of a 35-year experience with 2807 patients. Head Neck Surg 1986;8(3):177–84.

30. Renehan A, Gleave EN, Hancock BD, et al. Long-term follow-up of over 1000 patients with salivary gland tumours treated at a single centre. Br J Surg 1996;83(12):1750–4.

31. Maiorano E, Lo ML, Favia G, et al. Warthin's tumour: a study of 78 cases with emphasis on bilaterality, multifocality and association with other malignancies. Oral Oncol 2002;38:35–40.

32. Christensen RK, Bjorndal K, Godballe C, et al. A value of fine needle aspiration biopsy of salivary gland lesions. Head Neck 2010;32(1):104–8.

33. Tsai T, O'Brien JM. Masquerade syndromes: malignancies mimicking inflammation of the eye. Int Ophthalmol Clin 2002;42(1):115–31.

34. Read RW, Zamir E, Rao NA. Neoplastic masquerade syndromes. Surv Ophthalmol 2002;47(2):81–124.

35. Rothova A, Ooijman F, Kerkhoff F, et al. Uveitis masquerade syndromes. Ophthalmology 2001;108(2):386–99.

36. Cote TR, Manns A, Hardy CR, et al. Epidemiology of brain lymphoma among people with or without acquired immunodeficiency syndrome. J Natl Cancer Inst 1996;88(10):675–9.

37. Jahnke K, Korfel A, Komm J, et al. Intraocular lymphoma 2000-2005: results of a retrospective multicentre trial. Graefes Arch Clin Exp Ophthalmol 2006;244(6): 663–9.

38. Peterson K, Gordon KB, Heinemann MH, et al. The clinical spectrum of ocular lymphoma. Cancer 1993;72(3):843–9.

39. Akpek EK, Ahmed I, Hochberg FH, et al. Intraocular-central nervous system lymphoma: clinical features, diagnosis, and outcomes. Ophthalmology 1999; 1006(9):1805–10.

40. Brown SM, Jampol LM, Cantrill HL. Intraocular lymphoma presenting as retinal vasculitis. Surv Ophthalmol 1994;39(2):133–40.

41. Velez G, Chan CC, Csaky KG. Fluorescein angiographic findings in primary intraocular lymphoma. Retina 2002;22(1):37–43.

42. Intzedy L, Teoh SC, Hogan A, et al. Cytopathological analysis of vitreous in intraocular lymphoma. Eye 2008;22(2):289–93.

43. Buggage RR, Velez G, Myers-Powell B, et al. Primary intraocular lymphoma with a low interleukin 10 to interleukin 6 ratio and heterogeneous IgH gene rearrangement. Arch Ophthalmol 1999;117(9):1239–42.

44. Smith JR, Rosenbaum JT, Wilson DJ, et al. Role of intravitreal methotrexate in the treatment of primary central nervous system lymphoma with ocular lymphoma. Ophthalmology 2002;109(9):1709–16.

45. Wadhwa N, Vohra R, Shrey D, et al. Unilateral hypopyon in a child as a first and sole presentation in relapsing acute lymphoblastic leukemia. Indian J Ophthalmol 2007;55:223–4.

46. Hoang-Xuan T, Bodaghi B, Toublanc M, et al. Scleritis and mucosal associated lymphoid tissue lymphoma: a new masquerade syndrome. Ophthalmology 1996;103(4):631–5.

47. Doery SE, Clark BJ, Chrisopoulos VA, et al. Orbital lymphoma misdiagnosed as scleritis. Ophthalmology 2002;109(12):2347–50.

48. Gaucher D, Bodaghi B, Charlotte F, et al. MALT-type B cell lymphoma masquerading as scleritis or posterior uveitis. J Fr Ophtalmol 2005;28(1):31–8 [in French].

49. Demirci H, Shields CL, Karatza EC, et al. Orbital lymphoproliferative tumors: analysis of clinical features and systemic involvement in 160 cases. Ophthalmology 2008;115(9):1626–31.
50. Ferry JA, Fung CY, Zukerberg L, et al. Lymphoma of the ocular adnexa: a study of 353 cases. Am J Surg Pathol 2007;31(2):170–84.
51. McKelvie PA. Ocular adnexal lymphomas: a review. Adv Anat Pathol 2010;17(4): 251–61.
52. Chanudet E, Zhou Y, Bacon CM, et al. *Chlamydia psittaci* is variably associated with ocular adnexal MALT lymphoma in different geographical regions. J Pathol 2006;209(3):344–51.
53. Bhatnagar R, Vine AK. Diffuse infiltrating retinoblastoma. Ophthalmology 1991; 98:1657–61.
54. Shields JA, Shields CL, Suvarnamani C, et al. Retinoblastoma manifesting as orbital cellulitis. Am J Ophthalmol 1991;112(4):442–9.
55. Foster BS, Mukai S. Intraocular retinoblastoma presenting as ocular and orbital inflammation. Int Ophthalmol Clin 1996;36(1):153–60.
56. Shields CL, Ghassemi F, Tuncer S, et al. Clinical spectrum of diffuse infiltrating retinoblastoma in 34 consecutive eyes. Ophthalmology 2008;115(12):2253–8.
57. Grin-Jorgensen C, Berke A, Grin M. Ocular melanoma. Dermatol Clin 1992; 10(4):663–8.
58. Laver NV, McLaughlin ME, Duker JS. Ocular melanoma. Arch Pathol Lab Med 2010;134(12):1778–84.
59. Fraser DJ, Front RL. Ocular inflammation and hemorrhage as initial manifestations of uveal malignant melanoma. Incidence and prognosis. Arch Ophthalmol 1979;97(7):1311–4.
60. Yap EY, Robertson DM, Buettner H. Scleritis as an initial manifestation of choroidal malignant melanoma. Ophthalmology 1992;99(11):1693–7.
61. Kafkala C, Daoud YJ, Paredes I, et al. Masquerade scleritis. Ocul Immunol Inflamm 2005;13(6):479–82.
62. Palamar M, Thangappan A, Shields CL, et al. Necrotic choroidal melanoma with scleritis and choroidal effusion. Cornea 2009;28(3):354–6.
63. Wu J, Catalano E, Coppola D. Retroperitoneal fibrosis (Ormond's disease): clinical pathologic study of eight cases. Cancer Control 2002;9(5):432–7.
64. Vaglio A, Salvarani C, Buzio C. Retroperitoneal fibrosis. Lancet 2006;367:241–51.
65. Stone JR. Aortitis, periaortitis, and retroperitoneal fibrosis, as manifestations of IgG4-related systemic disease. Curr Opin Rheumatol 2011;23:88–94.
66. Kottra JJ, Dunnick NR. Retroperitoneal fibrosis. In: advances in uroradiology II. Radiol Clin North Am 1996;34(6):1259–75.
67. Thomas MH, Chisholm GD. Retroperitoneal fibrosis associated with malignant disease. Br J Cancer 1973;28:453–8.
68. Armstrong MB, Olson PR, Townsend RN. Gallbladder carcinoma and retroperitoneal fibrosis: a rare combination. JAMA 1989;81(9):1001–11.
69. Rivlin ME, McGehee RP, Bower JD. Retroperitoneal fibrosis associated with carcinoma of the cervix: review of the literature. Gynecol Oncol 1991;41:95–7.
70. Modlin IM, Shapiro MD, Kidd M. Carcinoid tumors and fibrosis: an association with no explanation. Am J Gastroenterol 2004;99:2466–78.
71. Gilkeson GS, Allen NB. Retroperitoneal fibrosis: a true connective tissue disease. Rheum Dis Clin North Am 1996;22(1):24–38.
72. Vivas I, Nicolas AI, Velazquez P, et al. Retroperitoneal fibrosis: typical and atypical manifestations. Br J Radiol 2000;866(73):214–22.

73. Moroni G, Gallelli B, Banfi G, et al. Long-term outcome of idiopathic retroperitoneal fibrosis treated with surgical and/or medical approaches. Nephrol Dial Transplant 2006;21:2485–90.

74. Adler S, Lodermeyer S, Gaa J, et al. Successful mycophenolate mofetil therapy in nine patients with idiopathic retroperitoneal fibrosis. Rheumatology 2008;47:1535–8.

75. Scheel PJ, Piccini J, Rahman MH, et al. Combined prednisone and mycophenolate mofetil treatment for retroperitoneal fibrosis. J Urol 2007;178:140–4.

76. van Bommel EF, Hendriksz TR, Huiskes AW, et al. Brief communication: tamoxifen therapy for nonmalignant retroperitoneal fibrosis. Ann Intern Med 2006;144:101–6.

77. Rho RH, Brewer RP, Lamer TJ, et al. Complex regional pain syndrome. Mayo Clin Proc 2002;77:174–80.

78. Taggart AJ, Iveson JM, Wright V. Shoulder-hand syndrome and symmetrical arthralgia in patients with tubo-ovarian carcinoma. Ann Rheum Dis 1984;43:391–3.

79. Fournier RS, Holder LE. Reflex sympathetic dystrophy: diagnostic controversies. Semin Nucl Med 1998;28(1):116–23.

80. Marinus J, Moseley GL, Birklein F, et al. Clinical features and pathophysiology of complex regional pain syndrome. Lancet Neurol 2011;10(7):637–48.

81. Stanton-Hicks M, Janig W, Hassenbusch S, et al. Reflex sympathetic dystrophy: changing concepts and taxonomy. Pain 1995;63(1):127–33.

82. Ku A, Lachmann E, Tunkel R, et al. Upper limb reflex sympathetic dystrophy associated with occult malignancy. Arch Phys Med Rehabil 1996;77(7):726–8.

83. Michaels RM, Sorber JA. Reflex sympathetic dystrophy as a probable paraneoplastic syndrome: case report and literature review. Arthritis Rheum 1984;27(10):1183–5.

84. Prowse M, Higgs CM, Forrester-Wood C, et al. Reflex sympathetic dystrophy associated with squamous cell carcinoma of the lung. Ann Rheum Dis 1989;48:339–41.

85. Derbekyan V, Novales-Diaz J, Lisbona R. Pancoast tumor as a cause of reflex sympathetic dystrophy. J Nucl Med 1993;34(11):1992–4.

86. Olson WL. Reflex sympathetic dystrophy associate with tumour infiltration of the stellate ganglion. J R Soc Med 1993;86:482–3.

87. Medsger TA, Dixon JA, Garwood VF. Palmar fasciitis and polyarthritis with ovarian carcinoma. Ann Intern Med 1982;96(4):424–31.

88. Cakar E, Durmus O, Kiralp MZ, et al. An unusual case of osteoid osteoma misdiagnosed as inflammatory joint disease and complex regional pain syndrome. Acta Reumatol Port 2009;34:670–1.

89. Summers CL, Shahi M. Epithelioid sarcoma presenting as the reflex sympathetic dystrophy syndrome. Postgrad Med J 1987;63:217–20.

90. Stamatoullas A, Ferrant A, Manicourt D. Reflex sympathetic dystrophy after bone marrow transplantation. Ann Hematol 1993;67(5):245–7.

91. Kiroglu MM, Sarpel T, Ozberk P, et al. Reflex sympathetic dystrophy following neck dissections. Am J Otolaryngol 1997;18(2):103–6.

92. Massard C, Fizazi K, Gross-Goupil M, et al. Reflex sympathetic dystrophy in patients with metastatic renal cell carcinoma treated everolimus. Invest New Drugs 2010;28:876–81.

93. Haan J, Peters WG. Amyloid and peripheral nervous system disease. Clin Neurol Neurosurg 1994;96:1–9.

94. Kelly JJ. Peripheral neuropathies associated with monoclonal proteins: a clinical review. Muscle Nerve 1985;8:138–50.
95. Rajkumar SV, Gertz MA, Kyle RA. Prognosis of patients with primary systemic amyloidosis who present with dominant neuropathy. Am J Med 1998;104:232–7.
96. Kang EH, Lee EB, Im CH, et al. A case of femoral compressive neuropathy in AL amyloidosis. J Korean Med Sci 2005;20:524–7.
97. Kelly JJ, Kyle RA, O'Brien PC, et al. The natural history of peripheral neuropathy in primary systemic amyloidosis. Ann Neurol 1979;6:1–7.
98. Tracy JA, Dyck PJ, Dyck JB. Primary amyloidosis presenting as upper limb multiple mononeuropathies. Muscle Nerve 2010;41:710–5.
99. Cohen AD, Comenzo RL. Systemic light-chain amyloidosis: advances in diagnosis, prognosis, and therapy. Hematology 2010;2010:287–94.
100. Palladini G, Merlini G. Current treatment of AL amyloidosis. Haematologica 2009;94(8):1044–8.

Index

Rheum Dis Clin N Am 37 (2011) 639–647
doi:10.1016/S0889-857X(11)00075-5
0889-857X/11/$ – see front matter © 2011 Elsevier Inc. All rights reserved.

rheumatic.theclinics.com

United States Postal Service

Statement of Ownership, Management, and Circulation
(All Periodicals Publications Except Requestor Publications)

1. Publication Title
Rheumatic Disease Clinics of North America

2. Publication Number
0 0 6 - 2 7 2

3. Filing Date
9/16/11

4. Issue Frequency
Feb, May, Aug, Nov

5. Number of Issues Published Annually
4

6. Annual Subscription Price
$282.00

7. Complete Mailing Address of Known Office of Publication *(Not printer)* *(Street, city, county, state, and ZIP+4®)*

Elsevier Inc.
360 Park Avenue South
New York, NY 10010-1710

Contact Person
Stephen Bushing

Telephone *(Include area code)*
215-239-3688

8. Complete Mailing Address of Headquarters or General Business Office of Publisher *(Not printer)*
Elsevier Inc., 360 Park Avenue South, New York, NY 10010-1710

9. Full Names and Complete Mailing Addresses of Publisher, Editor, and Managing Editor *(Do not leave blank)*

Publisher *(Name and complete mailing address)*
Kim Murphy, Elsevier, Inc., 1600 John F. Kennedy Blvd. Suite 1800, Philadelphia, PA 19103-2899

Editor *(Name and complete mailing address)*
Rachel Glover, Elsevier, Inc., 1600 John F. Kennedy Blvd. Suite 1800, Philadelphia, PA 19103-2899

Managing Editor *(Name and complete mailing address)*
Sarah Barth, Elsevier, Inc., 1600 John F. Kennedy Blvd. Suite 1800, Philadelphia, PA 19103-2899

10. Owner *(Do not leave blank. If the publication is owned by a corporation, give the name and address of the corporation immediately followed by the names and addresses of all stockholders owning or holding 1 percent or more of the total amount of stock. If not owned by a corporation, give the names and addresses of the individual owners. If owned by a partnership or other unincorporated firm, give its name and address as well as those of each individual owner. If the publication is published by a nonprofit organization, give its name and address.)*

Full Name	Complete Mailing Address
Wholly owned subsidiary of	4520 East-West Highway
Reed/Elsevier, US holdings	Bethesda, MD 20814

11. Known Bondholders, Mortgagees, and Other Security Holders Owning or Holding 1 Percent or More of Total Amount of Bonds, Mortgages, or Other Securities. If none, check box ☐ None

Full Name	Complete Mailing Address
N/A	

12. Tax Status *(For completion by nonprofit organizations authorized to mail at nonprofit rates)* *(Check one)*
The purpose, function, and nonprofit status of this organization and the exempt status for federal income tax purposes:
☐ Has Not Changed During Preceding 12 Months
☐ Has Changed During Preceding 12 Months *(Publisher must submit explanation of change with this statement)*

PS Form 3526, September 2007 (Page 1 of 3 (Instructions Page 3)) PSN 7530-01-000-9931 **PRIVACY NOTICE:** See our Privacy policy in www.usps.com

---

13. Publication Title
Rheumatic Disease Clinics of North America

14. Issue Date for Circulation Data Below
May 2011

15. Extent and Nature of Circulation

		Average No. Copies Each Issue During Preceding 12 Months	No. Copies of Single Issue Published Nearest to Filing Date
a. Total Number of Copies *(Net press run)*		1345	1300
b. Paid Circulation (By Mail and Outside the Mail)	(1) Mailed Outside-County Paid Subscriptions Stated on PS Form 3541. *(Include paid distribution above nominal rate, advertiser's proof copies, and exchange copies)*	500	444
	(2) Mailed In-County Paid Subscriptions Stated on PS Form 3541 *(Include paid distribution above nominal rate, advertiser's proof copies, and exchange copies)*		
	(3) Paid Distribution Outside the Mails Including Sales Through Dealers and Carriers, Street Vendors, Counter Sales, and Other Paid Distribution Outside USPS®	299	206
	(4) Paid Distribution by Other Classes Mailed Through the USPS (e.g. First-Class Mail®)		
c. Total Paid Distribution *(Sum of 15b (1), (2), (3), and (4))* ▶		799	650
d. Free or Nominal Rate Distribution (By Mail and Outside the Mail)	(1) Free or Nominal Rate Outside-County Copies Included on PS Form 3541	84	75
	(2) Free or Nominal Rate In-County Copies Included on PS Form 3541		
	(3) Free or Nominal Rate Copies Mailed at Other Classes Through the USPS (e.g. First-Class Mail)		
	(4) Free or Nominal Rate Distribution Outside the Mail (Carriers or other means)		
e. Total Free or Nominal Rate Distribution (Sum of 15d (1), (2), (3) and (4)) ▶		84	75
f. Total Distribution (Sum of 15c and 15e) ▶		883	725
g. Copies not Distributed (See instructions to publishers #4 (page #3)) ▶		462	575
h. Total (Sum of 15f and g) ▶		1345	1300
i. Percent Paid (15c divided by 15f times 100) ▶		90.49%	89.66%

16. Publication of Statement of Ownership
☐ If the publication is a general publication, publication of this statement is required. Will be printed in the November 2011 issue of this publication. ☐ Publication not required

17. Signature and Title of Editor, Publisher, Business Manager, or Owner

Stephen R. Bushing —Inventory/Distribution Coordinator

Date September 16, 2011

I certify that all information furnished on this form is true and complete. I understand that anyone who furnishes false or misleading information on this form or who omits material or information requested on the form may be subject to criminal sanctions (including fines and imprisonment) and/or civil sanctions (including civil penalties).

PS Form 3526, September 2007 (Page 2 of 3)

Moving?

Make sure your subscription moves with you!

To notify us of your new address, find your **Clinics Account Number** (located on your mailing label above your name), and contact customer service at:

Email: journalscustomerservice-usa@elsevier.com

800-654-2452 (subscribers in the U.S. & Canada)
314-447-8871 (subscribers outside of the U.S. & Canada)

Fax number: 314-447-8029

Elsevier Health Sciences Division
Subscription Customer Service
3251 Riverport Lane
Maryland Heights, MO 63043

*To ensure uninterrupted delivery of your subscription, please notify us at least 4 weeks in advance of move.

Printed and bound by CPI Group (UK) Ltd, Croydon, CR0 4YY

03/10/2024

01040444-0008